PRAISE
SHAME-FREE PARENTING

"Craig's work hits the true essence of parenting. You want to manage your child's development but realize you only have so much control over that process. He also hits on how stressful parenting is and that you don't have to repress your own emotions in the process. Given the modern cultural issues which face families, it's imperative to focus on resiliency and problem solving versus trying to protect children from every possible stress or emotional upset."

Michele Borba, Ed.D.
Educational psychologist and best-selling author of *Thrivers: The Surprising Reasons Why Some Kids Struggle and Others Shine* and *Unselfie: Why Empathetic Kids Succeed in Our All-About-Me World*

"A Must-Read for Every Parent!"
"As a mom, I've stumbled through the ups and downs of parenting, often feeling like I'm falling short or not doing enough. The idea of imperfect parenting gave me a breath of fresh air in the world of parenting advice, Instagram parents, and mommy blogs—wisdom and compassion shine through every page, reassuring us moms and dads that being a 'good enough' parent is not just okay; it's everything."
"I LOVE THIS BOOK SO MUCH!"

Lucy Murphy
Mother of two young ones

"Parenting has always been a gratifying but challenging responsibility. The challenges have intensified in today's world. The ramifications of such forces as COVID, political divisiveness, and social media have added to the stress and uncertainty experienced by children teens, and their families. Parents struggle with how best to raise caring, hopeful, resilient children in a stress-filled world. To assist parents with this struggle, Craig Knippenberg has written a very impressive book: *Shame-Free Parenting.* Not only does Craig describe the many issues facing kids and their parents, but he offers practical, realistic strategies for managing these issues. In addition, Craig's empathy for parents and their kids comes across on every page of his book, including his personal stories as a son, father, husband, and grandfather. This book will be a major resource for parents, teachers, coaches, and other childcare professionals who have the privilege of interacting with children and teens and helping them become more compassionate, self-assured, resilient adults."

Robert Brooks, Ph.D.
Faculty, Harvard Medical School (part-time) and coauthor of
Raising Resilient Children and Tenacity in Children: Nurturing
the Seven Instincts for Lifetime Success

"Craig Knippenberg has done it again! *Shame Free Parenting* is a solid follow-up to his first book, *Wired and Connected.* As a parent of adult children, I wish I'd had the benefit of Knippenberg's wisdom when I was raising my own kids. In his unique, easy-to-read, laid-back style, he assures parents that there is no need to be perfect! His words will resonate with parents of exceptional students as well. This book is full of practical advice for parents and reminds us that when all else fails, being kind is a great place to start."

Mark T. Twarogowski, MA
Head of School, Denver Academy

"I'm a mother of two boys, ages five and eight, and this book helped me immediately after reading The red light, yellow light and green light system has helped so much when it comes to disciplining my 8-year-old son. Understanding how his attitude, good or bad, affects the day, and how changing his attitude helps change his previous color for the better. Another helpful part of this book is about gaming. My boys love to play video games and there are several areas that help navigate how to create boundaries with healthier habits around how much time to allot them before sending them outside to be active. This book will be a book I will rely on for years to come. Especially with navigating the obstacles that lie ahead."

Amanda Scalbom
Craig's hairstylist and parent advisor

"Craig Knippenberg brilliantly gives parents permission not to be perfect and not to expect our kids to either. Parenting is an obstacle course, and this book does an incredible job of helping parents navigate obstacles in a practical way. As a parent of a neurodivergent child, I know how hard the journey can be. I often feel alone and isolated, and I am constantly judged as a parent. Craig's book puts everything into perspective! He provides a structure for parenting without guilt and shame and gives us a platform on which to allow for grace. Craig's years of experience working with children and families is easily recognized in his guidance, insight and understanding."

Cyle Feingold and Tiffany Feingold
Founders of Results Learning and Guiding Bright Minds and parents of an incredible neurodivergent child!

"As a parent and educator, I believe every parent and educator should read this book! Craig Knippenberg translates his vast knowledge of counseling, the social emotional development of children, and his decades of experience consulting with schools, into language that is 'parent friendly,' makes common sense, and is always optimistic. His advice is also very important for educators who interact with students for many hours each day. Based in research on brain development, Knippenberg has translated his ideas into advice that moves from practical ideas about routines, rewards, and consequences, to complicated issues such as social media, gaming, and smart phones. His insights address in practical ways the issues that parents struggle with as they negotiate raising children in today's culture. His wisdom, caring, and compassion for parents and their children are obvious, as he gets down to the business of empowering parents. As Craig says, 'There's only one parental behavior found in the research that will shape your child for the rest of their lives: *parental kindness.*' "

Judi Dodson, MA
Educational consultant

"What an encouraging, down to earth book! The title says it all. It shows that not only do you understand children and where they come from, but that you also understand their parents and the challenges they face in today's world. The book is well-researched, easy to read, full of realistic tips on how to create a positive family structure despite internal and external pressures interspersed throughout."

Susan B. Reid
Former MS principal, St. Anne's Episcopal

Shame-Free
Parenting

Building Resiliency in Times of
Hardship, Guns, and Social Media

Craig A. Knippenberg, LCSW, M.Div.

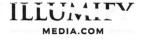

ILLUMIFY
MEDIA.COM

Published by
Illumify Media Global
www.IllumifyMedia.com
"Let's bring your book to life!"

Paperback ISBN: 978-1-959099-56-7

Typeset by Art Innovations (http://artinnovations.in/)
Cover design by Debbie Lewis

Printed in the United States of America

12/13/23

Michele,
Thank you again for your endorsement. It means the world to me. Blessings on all of your family adventures!

PS. Maybe we should go on a speaking tour together!

For my mother

For all the doctors, nurses, and first responders who were there for our family members during a global pandemic

For all the families in the world who found resiliency during and after the pandemic

Relax, you just have to be this side of good enough!

CONTENTS

INTRODUCTION

As Dr. Russell Barkley says, parenting is about you shepherding children, not engineering them.

I decided to start a podcast called *Legit Parenting*. It includes ten tips for surviving COVID, which I published in an article for the *Washington Post* in the spring of 2020. Those initial episodes, along with tidbits from additional episodes, form the basis for this book: *Shame-Free Parenting: Building Resiliency in Times of Hardship, Guns, and Social Media*. In it you will find timeless parenting and family strategies that helped the world during COVID and will help your family be more resilient through future tough times.

Currently, my biggest concern for parents today is the social media–driven frenzy about how you have to be concerned with almost everything you do with your children so as not to damage them or interfere with their successful trajectory into adulthood. As you'll see in chapter 1, this couldn't be further from the truth. While reading this book, I hope that you, as a parent, can let go of some of your stress, let go of guilt around past parenting decisions, and let go of any parenting shame you might feel from others around you.

As for the mental health of our children, it's not that today's parents are doing a horrible job. I see scores of parents every day who are doing an amazing job. My first big concern for the well-being of our children and teens is electronics and social media, which I address in chapters 4 and 5. While some parents are concerned about specific library books that might have a negative impact, children and teens are given access to some of the most heinous parts of human nature with a tool they can fit in the palm of their hands. Not only are they learning about these realities virtually, but many social media sites also teach your child or teen how to participate in the same behaviors. **Leave the librarians alone and focus on social media companies!**

My second big concern is the culture of guns in the United States, which I write about in chapter 6. Obviously, I didn't grow up with electronics or social media, but I did grow up with guns. Like the majority of dads in our Midwestern neighborhood, my father was a sportsman. We hunted small game and went target shooting and trap shooting. I received my first shotgun at age ten. My father taught gun safety to my two brothers and me, as well as how to shoot a gun, how to clean a gun, and how to store ammunition away from the guns. Never once did I hear my father talk about his guns existing for personal or home protection or the idea of using a gun against another person. I did the same thing with my son. As I inherited guns from my father, my son will inherit mine. I couldn't be prouder of that. I've also had many great adventures with my son when we've gone out to the local range. We once paid seven dollars a bullet on Father's Day to shoot a .50-caliber machine gun. It was a truly amazing experience.

Sadly, we now live in a country where scores of adults are settling scores with firearms, and millions of others are obsessed with assault rifles for personal and home protection and are even being prepared for armed insurrection. That fear is constantly being reinforced by our politicians, traditional media outlets, and social media. Others continue to extend the tragedy of Columbine High School by shooting more innocent children.

I have listened to children talk about their fears of a school shooting, or about the other mass shootings that are happening almost every day in our country. I truly believe that our founding fathers would turn over in their graves if they learned how many Americans are being shot down by their fellow Americans.

While COVID was tremendously difficult, and other ills such as racism and climate change are also very trying, it is social media and the proliferation and use of firearms that is tearing apart the fabric of our children and teens' mental health.

The Evolution of This Book

I've been a child therapist for forty years. I've been a consultant to schools, given national and international lectures, and published a book in the fall of 2019 that is based on a curriculum I developed for kindergarten through sixth grade to teach kids about their brains. It's called *Wired and Connected: Brain Based Solutions to Ensure Your Child's Social and Emotional Success.* The book is really about social and emotional behavioral development. It is written for parents, yet simple enough so that children can understand the concepts, and contains tons of parenting tips and activities for the whole family.

After the book's success, I was traveling and giving lectures while my therapy practice continued to grow; then the world just kind of stopped as the global pandemic hit. I decided to start a Facebook Live show to talk about parenting during the pandemic. My producer, Sydney, and I thought that the show would be going for a couple of weeks. We started the program once a week and then moved to twice a week. We hit two weeks, then four weeks, then four months, and then we hit seven months with no end in sight. At that point I thought, "You know, I'm going to turn this into a podcast, not just about the pandemic, but about how to be a resilient family." Given the rise in anxiety and depression in youth and adults, it's clear that times of hardship are stressful for the whole family.

The Crossroads of Shame-Free Parenting

Conceptually, resiliency really stands at a crossroad where three streets come together. The first street is your unique, imperfect child or teenager who has their own strengths and weaknesses and their own brain-based development. We have children with great impulse control and those with poor impulse control. We have emotionally even kids, anxious kids, angry kids, and depressed kids. We have children and teens who struggle with reading social cues and those who are social butterflies. We have students who use their empathy to build harmony with others and those who use their social abilities to attain power and control. This is all part of normal child and teen development.

At the second street in the crossroad is you, the parent. Your unique imperfect parenting style includes your strengths, your weaknesses, your emotional responses, and how you choose to exercise your parental freedoms. According to a 2022 Pew Research Center survey called "Parenting in America," while 80 percent of parents felt parenting was rewarding and enjoyable, two-thirds also said that it's harder than they thought it would be—including one-third of mothers who said it's a lot harder than expected. Today's parents spend more time and money on their children than previous generations and feel pressured to be more hands-on with their children. Sadly, many mothers felt judged for their parenting by other parents and friends.[1]

The third street is our modern culture. Prior to COVID, our culture was struggling with excess social media usage, increased suicide rates for our teenagers in 2019, school shootings, addiction to gaming, academic stress, worries about climate change, and online pornography. The social isolation of COVID spurned academic backsliding and record high levels of anxiety and depression among our children and teens. It created a mental health crisis that we are still trying to climb out of. These newer realities sit atop historical cultural issues like teen sexuality, drugs, alcohol, fighting, racing cars, and bullying. Then, you can add to that normal life and death transitions, and, for many, issues of poverty and racism.

The basic presupposition of this book is that you don't have to be a perfect parent at the point of all the crossroads. **Perfect parents do not exist. There is no perfect parent!** In the words of English pediatrician and psychoanalyst D. W. Winnicott, **you are good enough.** He believes, as do I, in the "sound instincts of normal parents."[2]

As you'll hear throughout this book, you have to be just this side of good enough. If nothing more, I hope this book will help you relax and remember that you don't have to do everything for your children.

The Goal of Every Parent

In my first book, I shared the ideas or concepts of Dr. Russell Barkley, who is the world's leading expert on ADHD. He is a phenomenal professor, writer, and author. He was addressing a conference years ago that I was attending about the concept of parenting, and he said, "Parents, aren't engineers; they're shepherds. You can't engineer a child."[3]

There's absolutely no research that says you are going to change your child's inherent genetic trajectory. They are who they are. There is a plethora of research that shows you can dampen down your child's trajectory in life. If you are neglecting a child, abusing a child, or not providing an adequate environment, then you can certainly affect the outcome of your child's future. But there is absolutely no research to say that if you're the super parent, you can turn your child into a super child through some type of super parenting strategies.

There's only one parental behavior found in the research that will shape your child for the rest of their lives: **parental kindness**. If you, as a parent, are kind to the postman, kind to the dry cleaners, kind the people at the restaurant, and, indeed, are kind to all the people you interact with day after day, then that makes you a kind parent, a kind adult, and your kids will become kind adults themselves. You are role-modeling empathy. While some of your guidance may stick, parental kindness is something you can pass on.

Your number one job as a parent is to keep your children alive. Then, you're giving them the basics. Every child needs a loving, secure, attached relationship with their parents or caregivers; adequate food, safety, housing, health care; an education; and reasonable boundaries. Throw in a sense of the spiritual or a sense of awe of something beyond themselves, and you've completed your job. Those are the things all children need. If you have those things, you're going to help them develop to their best genetic potential.

After that, you're just a shepherd. You're not engineering them. You're shepherding them to greener pastures. You are taking them to new places, new fields. You keep the wolves away, and you let them explore and choose to eat the grass they'll eat. You can introduce your child to all sorts of things, and you do not know what is going to take or not. Like a shepherd, you are just taking them around to different pastures and seeing what sticks.

My mother once said to me, "I used to think that you start to know how your kids would turn out when they hit about thirty, but, you know, it's really about fifty. You do not know how your children are going to turn out until they are about fifty." From a brain-based standpoint, she's right on because by fifty our emotions have settled down, and we have a little more impulse control, hopefully a little more wisdom, and we begin to see how our own children are going to turn out.

This is not to say we don't want our kids to be high achievers and accomplish great things. We all want that. One of my favorite words is *nachas*. It is a Yiddish word from the Hebrew word *nachat* that means "pride in your offspring." It's the pride we have in our children when we see them doing good things such as expressing empathy or maybe doing volunteer work. You have pride because your child is doing things that mean a great deal to you, but high achievement is not the goal of your parenting.

Your goal is to simply create or help develop a child who becomes independent and responsible while living in a community with others. Healthy, well-balanced children are those who are empathetic; work well with others; and are responsible, hardworking, and independent. They are resilient, which means they are able to handle life's pressures well. They can bounce back from adversity and remain even-keeled in all situations.

Being Resilient

Ultimately this book is about being resilient: having a resilient child, being resilient parents, and becoming resilient families.

It's not about happiness. It's not about your child being happy. It's also not about your child feeling high self-esteem. That concept has changed over the last thirty years. The founder of the self-esteem concept said that he invented it so children would be motivated to go out and serve their communities, express empathy, and help others to feel good about themselves. Self-efficacy is a better concept than self-esteem. I will address the differences in detail in chapter 8, but self-efficacy is about your child feeling they can take on life, meaning they can be independent, solve problems, and handle things.

Here is a story to illustrate the concept of resiliency. It was the day after Labor Day in Denver. We had an amazingly hot summer, and Labor Day was near ninety-five degrees. The very next day, a cold front came in, and we woke up to five inches of snow.

My wife and I are really into gardening. We love flowers. We went out to inspect the flower beds after the snowstorm, and, as you might guess, there were lots of destroyed flowers. All those beautiful, delicate little flowers were gone. But there in the yard, sticking its head up through the snow, was a bright yellow dandelion. It almost felt like it was mocking us. It was like the dandelion was saying, "Ha! You spent all that money and time on those precious flowers, and they died over-night. But look at me, I'm still here."

I let that dandelion live. Normally, I would take it right out, but I decided I'd leave that one. These are good times to be a dandelion family and raise resilient, dandelion children.

Being Good Enough

Finally, don't compare yourself to other parents and families too much. You have your own family story and your own unique intersection at those three crossroads of your child, you, and culture. You do need advice and other parents with whom to process your struggles, but make sure they are parents who listen and who understand what your family is going through, not those who try and tell you how to parent.

This book won't tell you how to be the perfect parent, but it offers strategies to help you be a good enough, shame-free parent. As stated by Dr. Spock in his epic book, *The Common Sense Book of Baby and Child Care,* "Trust yourself, you know more than you think you do." I couldn't agree more.

A good research study out of Pepperdine University explains how negative comments can eat away at your parental self-confidence.[4] They researched moms who were turning to online mom groups for ideas and support. On occasion, some would find worthy advice or might find another mom to learn from and aspire to be more like themselves. Unfortunately, they were also confronted by conflicting advice and judgmental comments. Rather than feeling better about their parenting, they felt worse. In fact, the study found that the longer women spend on mom-focused social-media sites, the higher their stress levels.[5] So, if you are feeling more stressed than informed and positive about your job as a parent, then get offline.

After all, relax, and remember, you only have to be this side of good enough.

CHAPTER 1

IT'S OKAY TO
LOSE IT SOMETIMES,
JUST NOT TOO OFTEN

I was asked to do a Zoom lecture for an international company in the fall of 2020. The title of said lecture was "How Not to Lose Your @#$% During a Zombie Apocalypse." Coincidentally, like many other parents, I had already lost my @#$% about two months into the pandemic. One of our daughter's eighth grade teachers called to say that she was grossly behind in her assignments and at risk of not graduating with her class. My interchange with our daughter was not pleasant.

The next morning, I apologized to her. I said, "Honey, I really want to apologize about how heated I got last night. I hope you'll accept my apology." She looked at me and said, "It's okay Daddy, we're all stressed from COVID." I wanted to ignite again over the missing assignments as the cause of this problem, but I bit my tongue and simply said, "Thank you." Fortunately, she buckled down at the kitchen table for the rest of the week for what we called "crisis schooling" and happily graduated.

To say that parents and kids were stressed by the pandemic would be an understatement. Being stuck together in the early months was hard, but we all hoped it would be over by the end of summer. The hopes were quickly lost as only some schools returned with in-person, socially distanced, mask-wearing cohorts and others barely went back the entire year. Teen anxiety and depression levels doubled in the 2020-21 school year.[1]

In May of 2021, Colorado health officials declared a youth mental health "state of emergency" as behavioral health visits to emergency departments shot up 72 percent compared with 2019.[2] Summer came with the hope of an open school year until the Delta variant arrived. While most were back in more "normalish" schools for 2021-22, there were clear gaps in the students' academic, social, emotional, and behavioral development. We continued to see the results of long-term stress—stress that was unrelenting for our children and for ourselves—and delays in development halfway through the 2022-23 school year. It would take an entire book to write about all the mental health problems we've seen during the pandemic. In reality, families really were not meant to have that much time together. All that time together and all that stress means that everyone in the family will probably lose it at some point.

During the pandemic, we hoped for the best for our kids' futures and for better parenting days ahead. Even when there is not a pandemic, we cannot forget that normal life has tons of stresses. Every generation has their own specific stressors. It was World War II for my parents and the Vietnam War, hippies, the race riots, and the Cold War for me. That's why focusing on becoming a resilient family is so important. However, you, as a parent, will not always be the picture of composure. And remember, you do not have to be.

What Does It Mean to "Lose It"?

What do I mean by losing it? Increased volume in reactions. Quick reactions full of emotional expressions and some poor word choices. You say and do things that later you think, "I really shouldn't have said that" or "That really didn't help the situation." I'm not talking about losing it physically.

Hitting or striking or pushing or grabbing your child in some way is not okay if you are hopped up on anger. In Colorado, and I don't know in how many other states in the country, corporal punishment (i.e., spanking of your child) is allowed by law. If you are a parent who chooses to use corporal punishment, it should never be done when you're out of control. You run the highest risk—particularly if you're lit and you start getting physical with your child—of hurting your child significantly. When you have Child Protective Services coming to your house, your parenting is way below good enough.

If you are going to use corporal punishment, it must be while you are in control of yourself. There is not a lot of research that supports corporal punishment as an effective deterrent or successful way to curb child misbehavior. Research has found that corporal punishment often makes a child's behavior even worse.

Your Temperament and Reactivity

If you are having frequent patterns of getting upset, yelling, screaming, saying hurtful things, jumping to conclusions, or getting physical, then you really should get professional help. If it is only sometimes, it might be helpful to look at your temperament and your reactivity patterns when under stress.[3]

Obviously, we all experience the gamut of life's emotions, but under stress, we tend to go to one or two default emotions. For some, it might be becoming more anxious about life and what's going on. Others might feel more hopeless or depressed. Others might get more irritable or angry. The key is to know which emotions you tend to default to so that you can catch them before they get away from you.

In addition to your temperament, there is also your reactivity level. Which is, how quickly do you react when stress happens? Some people are slow burners; they just kind of go and go until finally they blow up. Others might lose it right away; they get fired up and then they are fine two minutes later. For other people, the upset rises quickly, and they stay mad for a long period of time.

If you are in a situation where you cannot calm down and are close to really losing it, turn the situation over to your partner or simply walk away. Just walk away and get out of the situation. Go to your room, or the bathroom, and close the door. Every child behavioral specialist talks about the importance of children learning from immediate reinforcement, and while this is preferred, there is no problem in your family that you can't handle later when cooler heads can prevail.

Own It, Work on It, and Extend Grace

Emotional parenting means helping your child learn to respond in a "just right" (not too much and not too little) way. Many a young child has been helped with a sticker chart for exercising emotional control. That kind of behavioral approach can also work for parents. I've had numerous parents work on the same emotional system along with their child. A simple money jar or positive reinforcement system can work for both the parent and the child. Being a role model for your child means having insight into your own emotional reactions.

Given the rise in adult drug and alcohol use during the pandemic, I strongly encourage parents to avoid disciplining your child when under the influence.[4] Your judgment might be more reactive, and you are not going to have the self-control you need.

In addition to working on your emotions and self-care (see more in the next chapter, "Preserving Your Resources"), times of extraordinary stress call for the extension of grace to family members, friends, and those in your community. You do this by assuming others' best intentions. In her book, *Dare to Lead*, Brené Brown says, "I know my life is better when I work from the assumption that everyone is doing the best they can."[5] This relates, especially, to living in confined spaces with other people.

Let us say you and your partner decided that you really want to start having family-style dinners at the table and not eat in front of the TV anymore. You make the rule and explain it to the kids. Maybe a couple weeks later, after a very long and difficult day, you come in to find the kids eating in front of the TV. At that point, you might react to how your partner is not supporting the plan the way the two of you had agreed to. In this moment, you can think to yourself, "Is there another explanation or intention involved with this?" Then you can make a simple, non-emotional query about what's going on. It might turn out that your partner had a brutal day with the kids and knew that you had a tough day. She thought it best to have a nice quiet couple's dinner later.

We all have to extend grace and think about what underlying motivations and emotions might be driving another's behavior. Instead of reacting, be gentle in your response, be gentle with your voice, be gentle with your body posture, and be gentle with your queries. Kids especially often express their emotions with negative behavior and simply need a listening ear. (There are more tips on this in chapters 6 and 7.) Remember, we are all doing the best we can.

Letting Go of Parental Shame

If you do lose it, apologize and seek forgiveness. Apologizing means you own your emotional response, and you feel bad about it. You can own your feelings while also holding your child accountable for their behavior. For example, you could say, "I'm sorry I got so upset with you. I need to have better control than that. You will still have a consequence, however, for that offense." By the way, if your child shows the same maturity and takes responsibility for their actions, you can always cut the consequence in half.

The important part now is to forgive and forget, and let it go. Forget about you losing it, some other parenting mistake you feel you have made, or something you wish you had done differently. You have to give yourself permission to let go of your guilt and shame. It is human nature to link cause and effect with future outcomes, as if one bad parenting moment will have disastrous consequences for your child. **Parenting and child development is not about one specific moment but is more like a stained-glass window filled with thousands of moments that make up the parenting process. If you are a good enough parent, that picture is going to be fine. Give yourself permission to let go of guilt and shame.**

As a simple exercise, I often ask parents what they think was a big moment in their child's development (good and bad). I then ask the children the same question. Rarely have I ever seen the answers match up. The children bring up some obscure answer that parents do not even remember. In response to the parents' moments, children often reply that they were no big deal at all. Do not forget that we are all imperfect. Our kids are imperfect, we are imperfect, and you do not have to worry so much about the hard times. Someday, you will all look back and laugh about a few of these hard times at a family reunion.

In addition to forgiving yourself, extend grace and understanding to other parents. Misguidedly, there is a recent trend of parent shaming in our culture. Once you are a parent and have gone through enough hard times, you will understand how hard parenting can be and how unpredictable children can be. Parents who are judging other parents and children are living in a state of denial. They believe that neither they nor their child would ever do the things they are judging others for doing. That is, until they experience a moment that is below good enough or get a call from the teacher about something their child did. Now they have to eat crow and accept that every family has imperfections. While we have laws for parents who are below adequate, no good enough parent needs to be shamed by other parents.

If you are struggling with your own high expectations and want a humorous take on the topic of parent shaming, check out my interview (season 1, episode 20) of *How She Moms* podcaster Whitney Archibald.[6] She addresses how high expectations of parenting emerge from the pre-parent phase of life. During this time, we look at each other's parenting as a way to plan how we will parent someday. She has hysterical stories about moms who had big plans tossed out the window when the realities of actual parenting reached their doorstep.

As your children get into their twenties, they will engage in this pre-planning phase. In addition to looking at other parents, they will start to analyze you. What they liked about your parenting and what they did not like. When this happens, remember that they are pre-planning. Then say, **"Thank you. I appreciate that because it means that you are going to be a better parent than I was. I want you to be a better parent because we all must evolve and be the best, not perfect, parents we can be at this moment in time."**

Then, just wait another ten years when they are in the midst of parenting. That's when your children will realize how stressful parenting can be and that you aren't such bad parents after all.

A great way to support your parental self during all the years when you are parenting is with a parental gratitude box or drawer. Most of us had memory books of our infant's first year, which we tried to diligently fill out (often bagging it on the second or third baby). An easier thing to do is simply have a box or a drawer for your kids. When you observe them doing or saying something spectacular, write it down on a sticky note and toss it in. This could include comments from others on a report card or conversations you've had about your child when the other person gave you a positive word.

Recently, I randomly called a mother and left her a voicemail about how impressed I was with her fifth-grade son and his role model behavior during my annual puberty talk for the boys. On the last day of school, she came up to me and shared how touched she was by my gesture. She said, "I'm so glad I didn't answer the call and that I have it recorded!" While she can't put that in the box, perhaps she'll save the recording for a while.

Saving these memories will serve two purposes. First, pulling out a few of them on the day after you lost it with your child will soothe your heart and remind you that you aren't a horrible parent after all. Second, if you ever have time to do some journaling, you'll have a ton of notes to remind you of all the great memories.

Positive and Negative Reinforcement: Kids Need Both

Making things even worse for the average, good enough parent is the latest Instagram posts featuring glamorous, primped young moms who are promoting the "nothing but positive reinforcement for children" parenting movement. They offer several tips on how to prevent problems for your children and see all childhood behavior as related to the child's inability to express themselves appropriately. Nothing is seen as intentional by the child or worthy of negative consequences.

While the research shows that positive reinforcement should dominate your parenting, it also finds that using negative reinforcement 20 percent of the time is essential for civilizing children's impulses and emotions.[7] These relaxed Instagram moms promote the idea that all children's social brains are the same and that they are the same at all developmental stages. (I'm guessing they haven't parented a middle schooler yet or come close to understanding the difference between teaching a class of first or second graders compared to teaching much more mature fourth graders.) This is simply not true.

I have met a few children over the years for which a more relaxed approach might work. They have good impulse and attention control, a Winnie the Pooh temperament, and beautifully enacted empathy stemming from their well-developed social skills. For most kids, they need the parenting style that matches their poorer impulse and attention control, their moody temperaments, and their lower levels of expressed empathy. If you follow the Instagram moms' models, then 90 percent of parents will feel inferior because of how their unique children are responding to these unscientific tips.

How Much Control Do You Really Have?

As an infant, your child is completely dependent on you for their survival. You have control over their life. Every year they get older, however, your ability to direct their development decreases. The pressure on social media to be a perfect parent leads parents to think, "If my child is having a struggle in some area, it must be my fault."

A parent of an elementary student recently said to me, "What are we doing that's causing our children's emotional struggle?" I replied, "Nothing. It's just a normal developmental issue." What a burden for parents to carry around.

Much of the online advice is based on unlimited time that moms can spend monitoring their child's every behavior and short circuiting every misbehavior before it happens. Does that sound like your life? Even if you had the time, hovering over your children that much would be extremely detrimental to their development. Some of the best social development for kids happens when the parents aren't around.

At home, 99 percent of parents aren't dolled up or completely relaxed. During the lockdown, most of us wore the same clothes for days on end and our stress levels were at epic levels. I wonder how these social media parents would hold up trying to record their perfect Facebook or YouTube episodes when one of the kids comes running in, bleeds all over mom's dress, and is crying about being head-butted by their preschool sibling. It's hard to imagine how these online parents would live up to their own advice.

I do love the concept of mindful parenting (think before you respond), but it's not possible for any parent to be "mindful" 100 percent of the time. You are a person with your own needs and stress levels. We live at warp speed, and many parents can't find the time to use the bathroom most of the time. If you can pull off mindful parenting 51 percent of the time, you are doing well.

Perhaps the first and best writer and mentor on this topic is my former colleague Kristen Race. She was talking about this years ago and published her first book on the topic in 2014 (*Mindful Parenting: Simple and Powerful Solutions for Raising Creative, Engaged, Happy Kids in Today's Hectic World*). What I love about her work is that unlike the parent pundits below, she starts with you as the parent. By teaching you brain-based strategies for how to reduce your stress, you are then free to be more mindful in your approach. She doesn't just give you a list of dos and don'ts that you are supposed to follow. This leaves you feeling like a failure. I love how she says that mindful parenting can help you to "calm down" and "connect with your family in meaningful ways while making it fun!"[8]

Look out for quick and pithy posts on social media. One online pundit had a catchy pitch on getting rid of toxic phrases that are often used by parents. While I myself don't use many of them, I did think about how these statements (such as "children should be seen and not heard") are based on centuries of parenting wisdom and the reality of how difficult children can be. Children's behavior can be extremely irritating, and many times you just want a break.

In addition to pushing parents to be overly controlling, another Instagram reel talks about concern trolling when it comes to your children's behavior. Instead of asking your child about some concerning behavior, this social media mom says you have to avoid making them self-conscious or feel ashamed.

While you don't want to overdo your statements of concern, it is your job as a parent to monitor your child's development in many areas and address the concerns you have. As a tip for this important job, I often recommend phrases such as "It seems like..." or "I wonder about..."

Another so-called expert talked about how negative consequences teach kids to be sneaky because they don't know who they should express their needs to appropriately. Most kids know how to express their needs, but also know when you are going to say no to their demands. That's why they are sneaky. It's the classic "Mama upstairs, Dada downstairs" reenactment. If you don't like the answer from one parent, you run to the other to get what you want. Or as my three-year-old grandson said to me while I was loading him into the car seat for an adventure: "Mama says I don't have to wear my seat belt." Nice try!

Perhaps the most damaging idea being promoted on social media is that negative reinforcement will interfere with your parent-child bond. That's a total misunderstanding of the concept of healthy attachment. It's as if these online parents were listening to this line out of the *Love Story* movie: "Love means never having to say you are sorry." What nonsense.

Long-term, healthy, and attached relationships are built on a foundation of love that is then tested by the realities of real life and our poor coping skills. Parents get upset with their kids. Kids get upset with their parents. And parents get upset with each other. None of us, including our children, are perfect. To use the Swiss cheese analogy, we all have holes. That means you will get upset with your kid's behavior and will take action to prevent that behavior in the future.

This also means children should feel guilty about their actions and express remorse and make amends with those they have offended. It's your job to see that process takes place. Then you can hug your child, remind them how much you love them, and forgive them. That's the process for developing healthy bonds and attachments with your kids. The social media method of not having any negative reinforcement will leave your child fragile and vulnerable to any teacher or coach who reprimands them, or a future life partner who is upset with them.

While I agree that we don't want children to feel shame, there are circumstances for ourselves or our kids where that is the appropriate feeling. Acting in a deliberately mean and hateful manner is one of those circumstances. Don't be afraid to express your emotions because you are worried that you might hurt the parent-child bond.

Do You Struggle with Parental Inconsistency?

I do want to tackle the issue of parental consistency. For years, psychologists have been talking about how parents must be perfectly consistent with rules, consequences, and positive reinforcement. Consistency is number one. And indeed, research says if you had to pick one thing that would lead to child misbehavior, it is parental inconsistency.[9]

When parents are inconsistent it leads to problems in the family. You do not have to be 100 percent consistent. Being consistent 80 percent of the time in normal circumstances is fine. You really just have to be a B-level parent when it comes to consistency. If you are consistent 100 percent of the time, you'll put your kids over the edge, and you'll put yourself over the edge. In normal times, 80 percent is good enough, unless you have a preschooler (the age group that commits more acts of aggression per hour than any other human age group) or a teen. Then drop it down to 70 percent.

During the most stressful time of the pandemic, the definition of good enough parenting changed. During the lockdown, I recommended that parents shoot for 65 percent. If isolated with neuro-exceptional children (i.e., those with ADHD, mood regulation disorders, or autism spectrum disorder), preschool children, or teens, then 51 percent was just fine. It's 1 percent this side of good enough and maybe all you were capable of at that time.

Let's look at an example. Say you have a middle school boy whose feet have grown. His shoes are now size 12. And they stink, and he's constantly leaving them in the living room. Your family rule is that he is supposed to take his shoes to his room. If not, mom or dad is going to interrupt him in the middle of his gaming or homework, and he is going to be marching into the living room to pick up those tennis shoes. Pretty simple. So, 80 percent of the time, when you find those size 12 shoes, you should call the child into the living room and say, "This is not acceptable."

Now, let's say one night it's 8:30 p.m. and you're just beat. You've had a stressful at-home workday, have been dealing with the kids all day, and your preschooler is screaming and arguing. You find the tennis shoes, and you're just tired. You've already reminded him to pick up his shoes, and he keeps leaving them there. All you want to do is sleep. It's okay to just ignore the athletic shoes or to pick them up yourself and put them by his door. It's fine.

Shame-Free Parenting Tips for Consistency

1. Stick to your plan 60 to 80 percent of the time.

When setting it up, ask yourself, "Can I stick with any parenting plan 60 to 80 percent of the time?" You could create an incredible behavior plan and say, "Okay, kids, here's the new rules of the house," but if you, as a parent, cannot stick with it, then the plan is not going to work. Life comes in seasons with different ages and transitions that require changes in family rules, but if you can't hit 60 to 80 percent, don't take certain rules on. Let them go. There is no reason for you to keep knocking your head against a wall that you have built. Like your teenage son's shoes, just move them out of the way or let it go.

2. Use sticker charts.

When creating sticker charts for little kids, a problem with consistency appears when you forget about the desired behaviors you are trying to reinforce, can't remember to put the stickers on, or run out of stickers. I cannot tell you how many parents I have talked to over the years who got the sticker chart for their preschooler or first grader that didn't result in the desired outcome.

3. Create rules that won't stress you out.

As a parent thinking about family rules, you also need to ask yourself, "Do I want to do that?" and "Will it stress me out?" There is a lot of great parenting advice out there, but if it's not congruent with your life, the offered advice will not work. One decision that my producer, Sydney, and her husband made early on was that it is okay if there was a mess in the family room or wherever the kids' toys were because policing it was more stressful to them. They just accepted that kids are kids, and kids are messy.

To cut down on your stress, start by making a list of concerns that you have about your child. Then circle one or two of the concerns that you feel are the most important to improve upon. You must remember that many of these concerns will work out as your child becomes a social being. There is no better motivation to practice improved hygiene habits than negative feedback from peers.

4. Be mindful of different standards.

If you are a two-parent family, it's good that the two of you do this together and reach some mutual agreement of what you will focus on. While you can divide and conquer who will reinforce the various rules, you should both know what the rules are. (My wife and I have our own things we tend to notice more or are with our daughter more at certain times of the day.) Also, it is okay to have a few different rules when you are alone with the kids and your partner is gone. Like teachers at school, kids can get used to different standards. Don't let it get too far apart, however, or you'll hear, "But Mom, Dad lets me do that!"

CHAPTER 2

PRESERVING YOUR RESOURCES

When giving a lecture on how to preserve your resources, I had a PowerPoint slide of horses jumping off ancient sailing ships right into the ocean. A scene from the explorer Magellan and his discovery of the horse straights (a part of the Atlantic with little ocean current or winds) led to the question, "Why would the sailors be dumping their horses into the ocean?" They would certainly need them in any new land they encountered. The answer: the horses were drinking too much water—the water the sailors needed to get through this part of the journey.

In tough and uncertain times, such as the pandemic and the many other difficult life phases your family will go through, you need to preserve your resources as parents, especially your emotional resources.

The big questions in troubled times are: What resources can you hold on to and What resources do you need to let go of. And I'm talking about all sorts of resources. Obviously, I mean financial resources; there are many families in this country right now who are struggling to pay the rent or utility bills and put food on the table. In addition to financial concerns, there are also emotional, spiritual, and physical resources. It necessitates asking your family, "What do we value, what do we need to let go of, and what do we need to hold on to in all these areas?"

Parents need to be clear about these answers and then communicate them to their children. While you don't want to overwhelm them with adult fears, children need to participate in an age-appropriate manner and know about your resource choices. Not including them in an open and honest manner will introduce a host of unspoken anxieties into the family. Making some family decisions and bringing needs into the open reduces stress for everyone. When you follow your family decisions, it results in confidence and hope for the future.

Financial Concerns

For our family, we had to make both business and family resource decisions during the pandemic. My wife and I own one of Colorado's largest private mental health practices. Right off the bat, we saw an immediate drop (about 40 percent) in our revenue. The reason is that we specialize in group therapy for kids. Suddenly, we couldn't have in-person group meetings. So, we had to do some resource evaluation, purchase the necessary safety equipment for what could still be done in the office, and redesign our groups to be shorter Zoom sessions. Over the summer of 2020, we started back with in-person groups at half the capacity and developed a model that let us pivot between Zoom and in-person groups, depending on the status of the virus.

We also, as a family, looked at what we needed to do about our resources. I quickly realized that I didn't need to pay so much for dry cleaning because I was on Zoom most of the day. The gym memberships were put on hold along with eating out. I also gave up something I love: starting my day by reading two newspapers, then listening to NPR news, followed by checking online news throughout the day. About three or four weeks into the lockdown, I realized too much attention to constant news reports of COVID-19 was depressing me. It was just too much. I couldn't fall asleep. While I still read my newspapers each morning (stories that are delayed in time and lack the visual sensationalizing of TV or online news), I stopped listening to the news on the radio, and I stopped obsessively checking my news feeds. Trimming back stopped the depletion of my emotional resources and allowed me to be more present with my family.

We also decided to buy some weights for the back patio, return to our bikes, do some landscaping in the backyard, and buy a smoker. All these things were good for our physical and mental health and added to our resources rather than depleting them.

Talking to Children About Resources

Some issues around resources are above your kids' pay grade. After you and your partner have talked (or if you're a single parent, after you get your ducks in a row), then sit down with the kids and talk about what things they value, and what you, as a family, value.

Children love stories from the olden days, and they need to know that the current crisis that their family is going through isn't the first time in human history a family went through hardship, or is something their ancestors weren't able to overcome. To build a sense of family resiliency, start with a history lesson from your own family history.

For our family, we shared how our grandparents talked about the Spanish Flu, World War I, rationing, and Victory Gardens. My father often told stories about the Great Depression and how his family had to preserve their resources. This included a story about how he was disciplined by his mother for buying a nickel too much of hamburger from the local butcher.

For both my parents, World War II brought a need to preserve and utilize resources with care. Many did without the basics in order to support the war effort as they dealt with the losses of loved ones. My mother had to deal with the loss of her fiancé in the Battle of the Bulge, but she was still there to greet the returning soldiers at the train station just months later.

I also shared with my family how, when I was a teenager, we watched news programing of the Vietnam War and the military draft lottery, fearing that my older brother's birthday would come up and he would have to serve. Another crisis was the oil embargo when Jimmy Carter was President. We watched gasoline go from 20 cents a gallon to 50 cents, then 75 cents, and more. To preserve our resources, we drove a lot less and set household temperatures at 68 degrees during the winter and were constantly reminded to turn off the lights in the house. Even the movie theaters had to adjust their thermostats higher during the long, hot Midwestern summers.

Emotional and Spiritual Resources

After some history lessons, talk about what the entire family wants to preserve. For us, we wanted to maintain going to church. While our church was online for many months, we set up the laptop on the kitchen table each Sunday and served each other communion. As the church pivoted to outdoor services, we packed up our folding chairs and found a place in the shade. The outdoor Christmas service of 2020 under the stars on a warm Colorado night was one we will never forget.

We also enjoyed creating new adventures together. We bought our daughter a cruiser bike, and she started going on some bike rides with me. I go for long rides and my daughter was just starting out, so we would go as far as a little soda pop stand and a coffee shop. She would ride that far with me and take her book. Then she'd hang out for forty-five minutes, read her book, and have a soda pop until I came back for the ride home.

Obviously, the lockdown allowed families to spend much more time together. If you think about your lives before COVID, they were stressful. Children had multiple after-school activities, and teenagers had tons of homework. They were going here and there, and families were going at breakneck speeds. That kind of stress often leads to spontaneous explosions due to exhaustion and running behind schedule. The pandemic gave all of us a chance to slow down and spend time together.

At the same time, you had to decide, as a family, how much time you wanted together, and how much time you needed apart. Talking about this up front can cut down on someone feeling offended when someone says, "Hey, I kind of need a break just to be by myself." This need for a break is crucial for couples, children, and especially teens.

This is especially true for parents. You need a break from your kids to preserve your couple's emotional resources. My wife and I enjoy time together, just sitting, talking, and reading. During the pandemic, we established the five o'clock rule where she and I would head outside together and hang out. We loved it and our teen daughter enjoyed time to herself as well. While this might be more difficult to do with younger children, you'd be surprised at what kids can get used to when you make it a rule and start a new habit.

As a family, you'll also want to look at your social needs. People started talking about friendship pods as the initial lockdown began to lift. The kids needed to play with their friends, teens needed to hang out together, and parents needed to have some adult social interaction.

Early on, families found other families who had similar approaches to virus prevention and planned get-togethers.

Closely related to this expansion of social pods is your family's approach to in-person education. Families with health issues needed their kids to stay home with online learning while others were ready and raring to get back to school. Talk about these decisions in advance. While your children might not agree with your decision, it helps if they know the reasons why you are making it.

Physical Needs: The Need for Sleep

One of the most important resources you need to preserve for physical, cognitive, and emotional well-being is a good night's sleep. For younger ones, the first week or two of the lockdown brought about some fun, family sleep-togethers. For teens, the lockdown turned into late night gaming and connecting via social media, followed by sleeping to all hours of the morning. Neither of these are a good formula for getting the sleep each of you needs.

As the pandemic wore on, we saw more and more children struggling to fall asleep or waking up and coming into their parents' room three or four times a night. Maybe you experienced your child, who had been sleeping in their own bed, regress in their sleep habits.

As a parent, you can help your child make a connection between their feelings and this regressed behavior (see more tips in chapters 6 and 7). Help them see what is causing them stress right now by giving them opportunities to talk about some of their experiences at school or at home and what kind of anxieties they are having. You can then connect these emotions to sleep problems. They need to know how their anxieties affect their behavior. The key is *not* having this talk at bedtime.

In the morning, the brain wakes up from the lower areas to the upper areas. The last area to get "up and at 'em" is the prefrontal cortex. This area of the brain helps stop your child's emotions and then uses logic and reason to come up with solutions. At night, the brain falls asleep from the top back down to the bottom. For kids at bedtime, this means that the logical control area of the brain is powering off while their emotional brain (the area called the limbic system, located lower in the brain) is still on.

Many of your child's emotions are present all day long, but they don't rise to a conscious level. When they are actively laughing while playing, they aren't thinking about things that are frightening. During class time, the prefrontal cortex blocks out those undesirable emotions as they go about their schoolwork. When the prefrontal cortex shuts down at night, however, your child becomes conscious of those emotions loud and clear.

While we will talk more about structure for your family in the next chapter, you really want to set bedtime rituals through both the good and the bad times. During the early phases of COVID, it was easy to get out of the routines, and we saw how newfound sleep skills gave way to old regressive behaviors.

Shame-Free Parenting Tips for "I Can't Sleep"

As parents, you have probably experienced your child coming into your bedroom saying, "I can't sleep. Can I sleep with you?" If you are exhausted, it's easy to just let them crawl in with you. While that might work, it can also lead to some long-term patterns that are hard to break. Here are some tips that might work for you.

1. Consider worry jars, trouble dolls, and dream catchers.

Some children have worry jars, trouble dolls, or dream catchers to aid in the falling asleep process. The key is to close the gap between when your child is getting tired and when they actually fall asleep. As most parents know, if that gap gets too big, they can get agitated and it's going to take a while for them to calm down. I find it far more effective to talk about emotions in the late afternoon or early evening. Talking late at night can lead to endless conversations and the loss of sleep for everyone.

2. Say, "We'll talk about it in the morning."

When our daughter joined the family, she used to have a real struggle going to sleep because all these emotions would come up from her previous life at bedtime. I would just say, "Honey, we'll talk about that in the morning. I could give you the best answers in the world and they won't help, so let's save those for when your decision making is working again." To be honest, about 80 percent of the time, in the morning, she wouldn't even remember what she had been feeling the night before.

3. Decide alternatives for crawling into bed.

Instead of letting your child crawl right into bed with you, try taking them back to their bed and staying with them as they settle back to sleep. In addition to having a night light and favorite stuffed animal close at hand, you might also try a sticker chart or a positive reinforcement system for going back to their bed, or for remaining in their bed all night.

4. Try a sleeping bag.

If your child has formed a habit of sleeping in your bed and nothing seems to be working, there is the sleeping bag option. Place a sleeping bag on the floor at the foot of your bed so that your child is one step removed from your bed. Start with your child going to sleep in their own bed and do your bedtime routine. The rule is that if they wake up and need to come into your room, they can go to the sleeping bag but are not allowed to wake you up. After some success and plenty of positive reinforcement, you can move the sleeping bag into the hallway next to your door. The idea is to slowly get the child back into their own bed by giving them an option that makes them feel secure. On a much more serious note, the sleeping bag option can be invaluable if you have a teen who needs self-harm monitoring at night. Being close to one's parents at night can provide needed security.

CHAPTER 3

STRUCTURE IS YOUR FRIEND

We are creatures of habit and habits give us a sense of rhythm in life. Habits also free up brain space since you do not have to constantly learn new things. While we want to relax and live in the moment, by and large most of our time is spent directing our energy to accomplish goals. Structure routines to direct and channel your energy and your family's energy throughout the day and through the week to get things accomplished. As I love to say to my students, "Let's focus our energy please."

When you walk into any school classroom, you'll see posters everywhere about student behavior and the class schedule. Every day the teachers put on the board what the marching orders will be, what the class is going to do. Imagine the pandemonium that would ensue if your child went to school and the teacher had no rhythm, no class schedule, or no rules. It would be total chaos. Just walking into a classroom gives you the sense that this is where things are going to be accomplished. It's like hearing, "We are going to do some things for the kids today that put them in a mood for learning."

It's the same in my office. I have a special reading chair in the corner, and when I sit in that chair, I'm there to read. That's the only thing I do in that chair, and I love it. In the spring of 2020, during online schooling, we found that working in the bedroom was not a productive environment for learning for our teen daughter. It was not setting the tone for learning because everything else in her life is in that room. It became a dark hole. We moved her to working in an actual room in my office. She needed to wake up on time every morning, get dressed, and ride her bike to the office. This structure was much more effective and helped her get in a mood for learning. It is the same for your family; you need rules and routines to function and to get your kids ready to do things.

Creating a Schedule

At the start of the pandemic in March of 2020, Chris, a friend of mine who's a wonderful, widowed dad with a high school son and a middle school daughter, posted on Instagram his family's daily schedule. The chart went like this:

Wake up, family breakfast, dishes
Online school in separate spaces
Lunchtime together
Self-entertainment
Family exercise
All-house cleanup
Dinner and dishes
Family games
Bedtime

Like Chris, I suggest you have a daily schedule for your family. Plan chunks or blocks of time that fit into your schedule for every day or for the weekends. This is also a great idea to get through the long days of summer or through various school breaks.

Blocking out chunks of time to accomplish specific tasks is essential. We like to think that we can multitask, but to be honest humans do not multitask very well. The research on multitasking tells us that maybe 2 percent of humans can do it.[1] The rest of us are just running around, switching from one thing to another. Instead, create time blocks with specific tasks that have a logical order to them. Like Chris did above, you want to think in blocks of time in order to accomplish each task. This helps you from switching back and forth on very different tasks and wasting lots of time.

Starting out, it often makes sense to write down blocks of time for your children's school (from elementary school through high school) first. Then start adding in the blocks for the adults. These will be times for at-home office work, household responsibilities, childcare, and most importantly, blocks of time for your self-care.

For me and my wife, a daily time to work out was critical. For my mom, who raised five kids, time to herself was essential. Every morning after we had breakfast and cleaned up, she would retreat to the sanctuary of her bathroom and lock the door. She would spend thirty minutes in there every morning, reading her *Reader's Digest*. As kids, we knew we did not knock on that door unless there was an absolute emergency.

After you have created schedules for the house and family in general, help your kids add blocks of time to accommodate their responsibilities. Obviously, this will vary by the ages of your children. Elementary kids are going to be able to handle longer blocks of time while preschoolers need a much shorter block of time as their attention span is still short. If you have late middle schoolers to high schoolers, face the fact that they really want more control of their blocks of time. They want to be independent, so you must consult with them about the time they need for themselves and the time they need for school. Be realistic about the need to connect with their friends, either in-person or online, as well as blocks of time for family activities.

High schoolers especially are a different breed. Their personal plans for the spring and summer of 2020 were to pretty much sleep in, eat, make a mess, maybe complain, and go to their room for gaming or social media time. Rinse and repeat. For most parents, having a teen around the house with their no-schedule lifestyle drove us over the edge because we were so busy with our long lists while we watched our teens melting into their bedrooms. Although there are times when you need your teenager to be in their room to give you a break and allow you to get things done without the presence of a negative mood, teens also need structured tasks with prescribed blocks of time.

The planning for the age groups of younger children and high schoolers is particularly important because, to be honest, unless they structure their time, chaos enters their life.

Self-Entertainment

Most important for your survival and your child's independence, children need to learn to self-entertain. Some of you have kids who do that automatically. I was talking with a second-grade boy recently, and he said, "Yeah, I can self-entertain. I start to explore outside and just find all sorts of things." Other children struggle with self-entertainment and then they are on you constantly, saying, "Mom/Dad, I don't have anything to do!"

When I was growing up if I said that to my mother, she would retort, "Go find something to do, or I'll find something for you to do!" Those words meant chores. So, I learned to self-entertain.

The ability to self-entertain relates closely to the important topic of free play. Just playing without parent planning or hyper-supervision is essential for our children's development. All children around the world have an inherent desire to play. Early scientific theories viewed the function of play as learning survival skills. Recent research, however, theorizes something quite different. Rather than simply learning to physically fight, unstructured play helps children of all mammal species learn how to relate to each other so that they can succeed in a group as they get older.[2]

Children, while they are playing or learning how to negotiate, are learning how to cooperate. They're learning how to be with other humans because that's how humans survive. In addition, the physical contact that comes from kids roughhousing, doing each other's hair, or chasing and playing tag helps them learn how to bond with each other. That play and touch helps reduce cortisol levels (the stress hormone) and increases their oxytocin levels (the bonding hormone).[3] This chemical cocktail helps them survive with each other and adds to their resiliency during hard times.

Throughout the pandemic we had to make sure the kids maintained social distancing when they were inside. At recess, however, they found ways to play virtual tag, stick chase, and air tag. Thanks to lower cortisol levels from lots of physical activity, children were less stressed, happier, and ready to learn when they returned to the classroom.

During free play, children of all ages are also developing what is called their mirror neuron system. Mirror neurons are the brain cells that help us read others' non-verbal behaviors and conclude their thoughts and emotions (along with their verbal statements). These neurons help children learn how to relate and negotiate with others. In-person free play really enhances these opportunities. However, it needs to be done IRL (in real life) as the electronic world does not develop the mirror neuron system. (See the next two chapters for tips on adding structure to gaming and social media.)

In addition, free play increases prefrontal lobe development and functioning. When kids engage in free play, all sorts of logical thinking begins to take place in the brain. Free play also develops the ability to set, break down, and accomplish goals. Children who regularly spend time outside also show more empathy for others as well as exhibit increased confidence, social skills, and collaboration.[4] So, we want to focus on outside play to build resilient children.

Sunlight also helps your child produce the brain chemical serotonin. Serotonin helps us feel happy. In terms of the classroom, let's learn from Finland where students have the highest academic ratings in the world. Every child spends fifteen minutes an hour outside.[5] If you're worried about your child in the summertime running around with bare feet, research has found that running around barefoot is great for your child's immune system. It helps your foot microbes. Foot microbes flourish when there is contact with the dirt.[6]

Sadly, in the United States there was a 25 percent drop in free play between 1981 and 1997 and homework doubled.[7] Since the turn of the century, the loss of free play and increase in homework has only gotten worse. In 2011, American children were getting only twenty-six minutes of recess per day—including lunch![8] In the early 2000s, American teens were averaging about twice as much time on homework each day as teens did in the 1990s.[9] Kids today are getting even more homework while having less time to play. The post-COVID academic push has no doubt made this even more extreme.

There is also the relationship between less free play and increased fear-based parenting. I listened to an episode of the popular podcast *Freakonomics* in which author Stephen Dubner was talking about how, by and large, adults are pretty good at analyzing risk when it comes to something like our own safety behavior and how our investments might perform. Parents, however, are not very good when it comes to our kids; we tend to overinterpret danger and fear for our children.[10] And that makes sense for survival, but over the last twenty or thirty years, fear-based parenting has really taken off in this country. It's limiting free play opportunities. It's limiting the chance for kids just to be on their own.

Personally, I really wish we could ban the word *playdate*. When you use that word, it immediately implies who's in charge. It is the parents who are setting them up. The parents are figuring out who the kids will play with, when they will play, and where they will play. The parents are monitoring it. Instead, children should plan their own play and treat it just like recess. An adult can be out there on recess duty watching the kids to make sure nobody is hurt or bullying someone. But by and large, the kids should be on their own where they are free to play and have fun. Obviously, with COVID they needed some additional monitoring, but they still needed chances to just play freely.

I love Lenore Skenazy, the woman who developed the term *free-range parenting* after an experience with her own family. She was in trouble with the police for letting her nine-year-old son take the New York subway home from school, so she started a movement to remind parents that we need to let kids play, and that they need to be independent from us. She started a lovely program called the Let Grow Project. The program helps children become more independent. It is super simple. And it's all designed around letting your kid pick something they want to do. Maybe they want to cook dinner. Maybe they want to ride their bike to school. Maybe they want to take the dog for a walk around the block on their own. It is designed to help kids to be independent, to have time to play and to learn, and to grow and connect with other kids.[11]

House Rules

In addition to designing your schedule with blocks of time that include free play and plenty of self-entertainment for your kids, you need to go over the house rules and what the consequences are going to be if a rule is broken. I have always found success mimicking the school's behavior management system because children are used to it.

You'll also want to spend some time thinking about the house rules you want to have for different aspects of living with each other (roommate issues), as well as rules that will promote the values you want to instill in your children. My wife and I have never really pushed grades. That is not our thing. What we push is effort and being responsible. So, for our daughter, we have a responsibility check on Sunday night. We check to see if there are any missing assignments for the week and, if so, then the smartphone is gone for the next week. While some parents might choose to build behavioral standards around grades, we value effort and responsibility. Our rules and consequences at home reflect that.

Picking Up the House

There should also be rules about things that have to be done around the house and how your child takes care of personal items. In addition to having family harmony discussions (more on that in chapter 7), it's also helpful to have set consequences for noncompliance. If responsibilities are diligently completed on time and without being asked, then have some positive reinforcements for teens like increased privileges.

It is great to have structured schedules and set chores for children, but there are always problems around simply keeping the house tidy. The house got pretty pitted out when we were all in quarantine and also does during other times of family stress. The clutter at home can then result in more arguments and additional stress.

Start by not bringing up small issues all day long. Things like shoes being left in family spaces, a cereal bowl with a dry ring of milk, or the milk being left out are irritating, but they are not worth spontaneous battles that get in the way of what you need to accomplish. Instead, have a scheduled all-house clean up. Take a break and assign everyone an area to clean. Have some fun with it at the same time. Maybe it could be pizza and cleaning night on Friday nights. Remember, clutter can be brain damaging but not as much as constant arguing. **During times of hardship, just put the milk away and happily go about your day.**

Finally, as mentioned in chapter 1, when creating a system for your family, make sure it's one that you, as parents, can monitor and reinforce on a relatively consistent basis. There is no point to having an elaborate schedule or behavior system if you can't keep up with your own plan. Once you have your behavior system set, sit down as a family once a week to go over how the system is working and make any needed adjustments.

Shame-Free Parenting Tips to Help Create Structure

1. Use the red light, yellow light, green light system.

When my son finished first grade, I took the summer off, and we were just going to hang out together. I remember foolishly thinking that we would be free of the oppressive school year schedule, and I could just say, "Honey, what do you want to do today?" He would then answer, "Let's go for a hike/swim/build sandcastles." I thought it was going to be fabulous! It was a nightmare. Every morning, after we'd had breakfast and enjoyed twenty minutes of reading time up in the tree house, I'd ask what he wanted to do. The standard grumpy reply was, "Nothing!"

After a week, I decided to bag that system and instead created a weekly schedule of what we would be doing. I also added the red light, yellow light, green light system from his school. I cut out a card of each of the three colors. Every morning, my son would start with a green card up on the fridge. His goal was to keep the color on green by maintaining a positive attitude and cooperating with the rules. If he had a lapse in behavior, the yellow warning card went up. If he made amends, it went back to green. If the undesirable behavior continued, it would turn to red, and he'd have a consequence. We also set a goal for the number of green card days that he could achieve for the rest of the summer, where he could earn a trip to the local fondue restaurant (his favorite). He achieved the goal, and it ended up being a great summer.

2. Make to-do lists.

You can also make a small to-do lists for your kids every day. My wife is big into that. She writes out a sticky note for our daughter every morning that has a list of things, such as emptying the dishwasher or taking the dogs for a walk. The list has just some basic things that need to be accomplished that day.

3. Be calm, consistent, and concrete.

Walk into any elementary school classroom and you'll see the schedule for the day and the rules of behavior listed on the board. These are very specific, concrete rules that are applied consistently each and every day. Having those two factors clearly displayed allows the teacher to calmly manage the students throughout the day. While some issues always arise that might rattle the teacher's calm composure, not having the consistent or concrete rules would create chaos.

For additional ideas on behavioral reinforcement charts, homework routines, organization, motivation, and independent responsibility taking, check out: Wired and Connected.

CHAPTER 4

STRUCTURED GAMING

Several years ago, prior to the pandemic, I was asked to do a lecture for parents and their children and teenagers in Evergreen, Colorado, on the topic of how gaming and social media impacts the brain. I created a role-play exercise where students acted out different parts of the brain that function while they're gaming. One of the students, about age ten, was in the hot seat. He was the gamer. All the other students stood behind him, and I directed them on what to say as different parts of the brain.

At one point, as the narrator, I turned to a lovely woman in the front row, one of the moms, and said, "Bob is playing, and it's been forty-five minutes. What do you do?" His lovely mother said, "Honey, it's time to turn off the machine." I took the microphone up to Bob and out of his ten-year-old mouth came, "Shut up, mom."

The audience was just stunned. I was stunned. The only thing I could think was "Whoa!" I looked at everybody and said, "Welcome to family night in America. This is happening everywhere in the country every night." If you've ever had the same experience, then this chapter is for you.

I'll show you how to solve the problem. First things first: you have to have structure around electronics and social media, which have become a huge problem for families. Given the amount of content on this subject, we will tackle gaming in this chapter and social media in the next chapter.

A 2021 article in *The New York Times* mentioned that the longer kids have been playing, the more likely they are to develop a habituated behavior, and the harder it is going to be to break that habit. In other words, during COVID, the genie got out of the bottle, and we need to get it back in. The app called Roblox, for example, averaged 31.1 million users a day during the first nine months of 2020; that's an increase of 82 percent.[1] The statistics on this one app is just a snapshot of the increasing number of children who are captured by electronic gaming.

Another specialist said this whole COVID thing has been a gift to the game makers. They have a captive audience. The cost will be borne by our families because increased online use is associated with anxiety, depression, obesity, aggression, and addiction to the medium itself.[2]

The Positive and Negative Effects of Gaming

I'm not an anti-gaming person. Researchers have even found some positives that go along with gaming, and I will explain how this works in the brain as the chapter unfolds. Here is the good news: twenty minutes of gaming relaxes your brain.[3]

There is also some research that concludes families who game together (parents with their children) are actually closer as a family.[4] This makes sense because as parents you are entering your child's world.

When you play the game with your children, they are teaching you. They feel like you're in tune with their world.

In March of 2020, when the lockdown began, I recommended that parents stretch my normal suggestion of allowing kids thirty to forty-five minutes a day of gaming during the week to maybe double that. I thought, "Let's give them two hours a day because, to be honest, parents need a break." All parents need breaks from their children no matter their age.

Unfortunately, gaming time turned into nine to ten hours a day as the pandemic wore on. After students returned to school, it was time to go back to normal gaming standards. My recommendation is thirty to forty-five minutes a day on school days (perhaps an hour for older teens) and two thirty- to sixty-minute blocks on weekends that are separated by an hour of "in real life" (IRL) activities.

During the week the block of gaming time should be done after homework and chores are completed. While this is my standard recommendation, I also have some students who benefit from a block right after school to help them unwind from the day's stress. That's okay, as long as the device is getting turned off on time and the aforementioned tasks are being completed.

Looking at the negative side of gaming, Dr. Michael Rich from Harvard Medical School's Center on Media and Child Health says, "Boredom is where creativity and imagination take place."[5] Today's students, driven even further into boredom by the pandemic, are used to constant stimulation from the outside world and, thus, are less likely to turn inward as a source for inspiration and creativity.

The Brain's Attraction to Gaming

To help understand why gaming is so attractive, I'm going to try to help you understand how your child's or teen's brain functions. For starters, never forget that there is a huge difference between the child brain and the teen brain, and, yes, the adult brain.

At the top part of the neck is your brain stem, which is made up of the midbrain. The thalamus, at the top of the brain stem, receives all the sensory input (except smell) that comes into the brain. The midbrain is the place where our brains produce a variety of neurochemicals that are literally hijacked by the design of electronic games and social media apps.

One of the neurochemicals is called dopamine. There are two pathways that the dopamine travels: one regulates physical movement and the other one goes up to the limbic system (think of a donut surrounding the brain stem) where our brains produce the many emotions that humans feel. The dopamine pathway, or highway, goes right to the area of the limbic system that processes the feeling of desire. It also passes through the part of the brain that is wired for novelty. When humans find something new, we want to check it out further and hope for a pleasurable reward. We're constantly searching for new things. The phrase I love is: *We are always looking for that shiny nickel instead of completing the more mundane tasks at hand.*

This desire, novelty, and reward system is critical for our survival. It motivated our ancestors to find food, procreate, and engage in other survival instincts. While dopamine juices the system, our brain's pleasure "hot spots" may or may not be activated by pursuing the desire.[6] For example, if you eat a fabulous meal, your desire for food is satiated, and you'll have a sense of pleasure. If the meal isn't very good, you'll take care of your desire, but not feel the pleasure system light up. As my mom used to say, "Hunger is the best cook!" When you think about how many children or teens find great pleasure in junk food, you can see that trying to satisfy their desire for food with healthy choices can be difficult.

After cutting through the desire, novelty, and reward area, the dopamine highway travels up to the front part of our brains (think of your forehead). There are two areas of the frontal lobe to which the dopamine travels: the lower region is responsible for impulse control while the upper part is responsible for what are called our executive functions (i.e., attention, organization, working memory, and time management).

The frontal lobe in humans is more developed when compared to other species. In *Wired and Connected,* I call this area the President as it's where we can learn to stop before we react and engage logic and discipline as we complete life's tasks. (*Wired and Connected* does a deep dive into all these executive functions and provides strategies for enhancing your child's brain development.)

When this dopamine system is working at optimal levels during our day, we try and find some desire in our daily tasks. Our impulse control is engaged when we are doing something else that might be more enjoyable, or when we are acting in a socially inappropriate manner. It helps us to organize and plan what we are doing, stay on task as we remember the various steps that need to be done, and perceive and manage time so that we can move on to other matters.

Obviously, this is all much easier when we are doing things we like. Remember the classes you dreaded versus the classes that filled you with joy, curiosity, and excitement? In these later instances, our dopamine levels rose higher and we wanted to focus even more in those classes.

For our ancient ancestors, finding sweet berries and fruits gave them an extra juice of dopamine, which signaled the brain to focus on the berries and hunt for more. When it comes to the design of electronic games, this same ancient system for desire, novelty, and anticipated reward is utilized to keep the participant engaged for as long as possible.

Like a casino, the games are made to be fun and exciting with all sorts of new possibilities (things like air drops, new weapons, or extended health) randomly appear, and the player can go right for them. Players can also compete with their friends and show off their score or buy new outfits for their avatar with the simple input of a parent's credit card information.

Hyper-focus

As the player's dopamine levels soar even higher (some first-person shooter games can increase dopamine levels sixteen times their normal levels—the same as marijuana), the desire and novelty systems are lit up. The extra dopamine then hits the upper President with the message PAY ATTENTION. This is otherwise known as a state of hyper-focus.

Other areas of the frontal lobe are dampened as the player loses track of time, completely forgets that homework or chores need to be done, and can't stop their impulse to play even more. That is how you get a kid to scream "Shut-up!" or "I just need to get to the next level!" or "I can't let down my friends—they will hate me!" to their frustrated mother.

By the way, the next time your child says, "My time isn't up; I just started," they really do think that because their time management system is shut off. That's why both children and adults chronically underestimate the amount of time they spend on their devices (by 20 percent on average).[7] In addressing the problem, make it a family affair. Have everyone track their time on their devices for a week. Then discuss appropriate limits for everyone in the family.

One of the keys for helping your child manage gaming is to understand that there is this tiny window that exists between the normal baseline of dopamine levels and extreme hyper-focus. You are probably familiar with the concept of single-mindedness or getting into a flow. This happens when we are doing something we really like and are focused on that one task. This might be meditation, exercising, or completing a jigsaw puzzle. As mentioned earlier, when it comes to gaming, twenty to thirty minutes can relax the brain. It can leave you feeling refreshed and ready to move on to other tasks. However, after thirty minutes of electronic use, the dopamine levels continue to rise and put you into the hyper-focused state.

The Emotional Aftereffect

The other piece parents must handle is the emotional aftereffect. First, you have to fight the desire circuit just to get your kids off the device. After you finally get them off the game, they're just plain irritable or moody for an hour or two afterward. That's a side effect from the dopamine levels plummeting after playing for too long. Sometimes they'll plummet even lower than they were before they started gaming. That means your child's ability to be diligent with their studies or a chore is completely gone. You might also find them sneaking around for more screen time.

Consideration must also be given to the teen brain. Dopamine levels in the teen brain naturally drop in half when their President is being completely redesigned. This means that they are naturally more spacey and disorganized. It also means that they become bored very quickly. This boredom turns them into stimulus junkies. They're looking for action all the time and become risk takers. For a teen, the idea of borrowing their dad's convertible and driving down the highway at 90 mph with their passenger standing up seems like a fun thing to do.

Too often, this thrill-seeking means that teens turn to gaming. Rather than writing or reflecting and having more creative thoughts it's far easier and more rewarding for many teens to just jump onto their electronic devices.

Electronic Games at Nighttime

Finally, I want to talk about the nighttime usage of electronic games. If you want to create a sleep disorder for your kid, let them game nonstop right before they go to bed. There are several harmful factors with gaming before bed.

The first has to do with the emission of light coming from the device. Most devices produce blue light waves, which wakes up the brain. Our ancestors woke up and got active as the sun rose and the sky turned blue. As the sun sets, we are washed over with yellow light. The yellow light rays cause the brain to produce melatonin, which triggers our brain to fall asleep.

Gaming an hour or two before bedtime stimulates the brain to wake up and delays the release of melatonin. After gaming, your child can't fall asleep for several more hours. If they do fall asleep, research finds that all the movement on the screen makes for a restless sleep.[8] This is not the kind of restorative sleep the brain needs. While I recommend no electronics at least an hour or two before bed, make sure the device is set to a nighttime setting. While all the movement is still there in the action of the game, the light rays being emitted will be more yellow. Come winter, when there is less daylight, make sure the nighttime settings are on.

The other aspect of gaming and sleep disturbance relates to violent action on the screen (most notorious in first-person shooter games). First-person shooter games produce the stress hormone cortisol. While playing, the brain does not know that it is playing a video game. It actually responds to the game as if it were a real-life struggle for survival.

This perception tells the amygdala (the fight or flight response area of the brain located next to the thalamus) to produce cortisol. Cortisol floods the body and directs blood flow to arm and leg muscles, causing them to tense up. It quickens the heart rate and breathing and shuts down digestion. Even when finished playing, it takes time for the cortisol to process out of our systems, and it tells the brain to etch into memory everything that happened while playing. This isn't a good recipe for good health or a sound night's sleep, or for focusing on homework.

Warning Signs of Electronic Overuse

Parents often ask me about the troubles of too much gaming or screen time. You want to look for the warning signs that are based on research and common sense. One obvious warning is if your child is having a hard time getting off their device, and it turns into an ugly fight every night. Family time is supposed to be made up of fun experiences together. Playing a game or even watching a favorite TV show together is much better than everyone retreating to their rooms (parents included) and getting on their devices.

Steadily Needing More Game Time

The constant addiction to gaming and the need to increase the amount of time is no different than the alcohol or drug addict who needs increased quantities for the same desire and reward sensations. When dopamine repeatedly floods the brain, the brain will regulate itself to decrease the amount of dopamine being released. In order to maintain that desire or novelty rush, the player needs to spend more time on the device.

If your gamer needs increasing gaming time to get their dopamine juice, there is a problem that needs to be discussed. Parental authority is also needed to fight the budding addiction. Stealing cookies from the cookie jar does not mean your gamer has a horrible problem, but if they're repetitively doing it or are running up charges on your credit cards, then you have a serious problem.

Increasing the Level of Intensity of the Games

The brain likes novelty. After a while, with any game, the brain gets bored, and the gamer wants to move on to something new and more spectacular. This is a normal side effect; however, if your gamer is really craving something new all the time and going to extremes with intensity and cost, then that is a concern that needs to be addressed.

Only Being Able to Relax with Gaming

As parents, you might have a cocktail in the evening to relax after a difficult day. If that's the only way you can unwind, however, you are in for some longer-term problems. Parents must also be able to demonstrate multiple ways to handle a bad day, such as exercising or reading a book. Movement is great for stress relief: you can go for a walk, play with the dogs, or play with your children. If gaming is the only thing that makes your child or teen feel better, then that's a warning sign of problematic behavior.

Obsessive Thinking

If gaming is all a gamer can think about when they are not playing, you could have a problem. That said, we all know that children can be amazingly obsessive with their passions and hobbies. You can try talking to your child about other aspects of life or get them involved in other IRL activities. Participating in another activity can also be the golden ticket for earning gaming time.

Social Isolation

If your gamer is becoming more socially isolated, then you might be facing a bigger problem. Rules on gaming were greatly relaxed during the pandemic (or other family times of hardship), but now it's time to reclaim your standards. If you see that your child no longer participates in sports or hobbies and academics are going down the hill, it's time for a change.

Obviously, if your child is not exercising and becoming obese from gaming or if they're soiling their pants because they can't take a break to go to the restroom or they refuse to come out of their rooms for family dinnertime, then you must trim it back. Whatever the reason is for trimming back gaming time, remember that you will get lots of "noise" from your child in return. Parenting means dealing with noise after your decisions. A good mantra for your kids is *Everything in moderation*.

Managing Gaming, Smartphones, and other Devices

It is getting tougher to monitor gaming with the current generation of smartphones compared to the old days when parents could shut the router off. With smartphones and school laptops, children and teens find ways to game that you or your school's IT director never thought possible.

In our house, our daughter, even at age seventeen, still has to bring her phone into our bedroom when she retires for the night.

(Fortunately, she's very quiet when she comes in at eleven o'clock when we are already fast asleep.) When she was younger, we would charge her laptop in our room. My advice is to take the devices.

If you leave devices in your child's room, then you are creating severe temptations, and children can be very creative. Children and teens (so called digital natives) know plenty of ways to discover your parent password and shut off or alter the most secure of parent protection networks. As one third grader said to me, "There are lots of temptations online and some kids know their parents' passwords."

Contrary to the idea that kids are sneaky only because they don't know how to express their needs, this statement reflects how children are sneaky because they want things, and they haven't developed the ability to manage their brain-based impulses. Sadly, our children and teens now have temptations that our ancestors were never exposed to.

One of my favorite articles on the topic of children and teens being sneaky with electronics provides several techniques that kids used to hack their parents' control systems, including changing time zones, tapping on "Ignore Limit," redownloading an app, screen recording to steal your password, downloading software that bypasses limits, and turning to a burner phone.[9] In old-fashioned terms, it's the cops trying to keep up with the robbers.

If you think your kid is only doing schoolwork on their school iPad at night, you may need to take a second look because your child or teen can switch screens quicker than the blink of an eye. If they hear your footsteps in the hall, they're back to the school site before you can check. That's why many parents require computer schoolwork to be done in public spaces. The right to be in one's room alone with a device should be earned by trustworthy behavior.

How can you keep things healthy? First, try some online games with your kids. Play for twenty to thirty minutes and then turn it off.

As you read the tips below, keep in mind your child's social brain configuration. In general, children and teens with good self-control and a strong moral and ethical drive, or students who don't care about gaming, don't need the rules to be too strict.

If your child is the opposite, the rules need to be stricter. Believe it or not, I've had some students who were actually using screen time to explore educational content (a junior just told me about the streaming service Curiosity and all its great brain programming). For many others, however, this is just an excuse to game longer.

In addition to setting limits, you might also want to seek professional guidance. Kids generally seem to understand things better when I talk about what's going on in their brains in a relatable way. If your child has social anxiety or a social processing disorder (such as autism), then they will be particularly vulnerable to overdoing electronics. For many, the computer becomes their private world where they feel relaxed and secure. To understand why they might need more computer time, consider individual or social development group therapy. Our social development camps have been booming the last several summers.

Shame-Free Parenting Tips to Help Manage Gaming

1. Establish rules for acceptable lengths of time.

For students in lower school, aged kindergarten through fifth grade (sixth grade maybe), do not allow gaming at all during the school week, or do one block of thirty minutes on one weekday only. Emphasize getting homework and chores done first. The decision about no gaming during the week is up to you. You get to pick and choose because it is your child. Don't feel shame or guilt about your decision, and it doesn't matter what other parents are doing.

With any game rules you establish, make sure it's not within an hour of bedtime and reinforce that gaming must stop when you say stop. If your child doesn't get off after a five-minute heads-up, then they lose their gaming time for the next day. Weekends could be two blocks a day with an hour block between for some good old-fashioned fresh air.

For older teens—seventh grade through tenth grade—you can expand to forty-five or sixty minutes a day and two blocks on the weekends, provided that grades and chores are up to standards.

For eleventh and twelfth graders, I strongly recommend you give them the freedom to set their own limits and then reestablish more stringent limits if they aren't being responsible. I've known several guys who failed their first year of college because they never learned how to put limits on themselves. Gaming all night and sleeping through classes is not a recipe for success.

2. Create a budget for gaming.

Talk about how much money your child or teen can spend on the games and all their exciting upgrades. You should definitely have a rule or a limit on how much they're allowed per month on games and from whose pocket the money comes. I always prefer that children and teens spend their own money. If you find out that they have used your credit cards for purchases, then cut off all access. Once you have a new credit card, make sure not to leave it lying about.

3. Find age-appropriate electronic games.

For the younger ones, I'd be very cautious about the first-person shooter games. I'd also talk to them about only playing with IRL friends in a private gaming room. If you allow them to play in public games, your fourth or fifth grader could end up being victimized by someone they thought was another kid. If they play with teens, your younger child will be exposed to words you never wanted them to know. Instead, find games that increase language and cooperative social development.

4. Set limits.

When setting limits, it's common to have two parents who do not see eye to eye. Both parents need to suggest their desired limits and then cut it in the middle. That also includes an agreement that each parent will stick to these limits at least 85 percent of the time. After all, there could be a special bonding moment when you and your child binge on some gaming time together. That's no different than letting them stay up late for a sporting event. Just don't do it all the time.

I also have stories from numerous parents who pulled their kids totally off gaming for a set period of time and came back a couple of weeks later saying, "It's like my kid has come back. They were so upset at first but now they are happier again."

5. Create a gaming community.

Finally, don't hesitate to talk to the parents of your child's friends about their standards and rules. One of the legit complaints for kids during COVID was that their friends played at different times than they were on. While this was sometimes manipulative, it was also true and interfered with group-based gaming. After my school lecture on this topic, one creative group of parents all agreed to have the same group gaming hour. Brilliant! It takes a village to raise a child.

CHAPTER 5

TIKTOK GENERATION

Has your family been taken over by social media? In this chapter, we will be exploring social media and how you, as parents, can start to take back control. We will first look at the depth of this crisis with our older children or teens and then look at how social media apps, such as TikTok, have literally hijacked different areas of the brain. The chapter concludes with the strategies and appropriate structures to embrace the positives of social media while decreasing the negative impacts.

The Positive and Negative
Effects of Social Media

As I mentioned in the previous chapter with electronic gaming, there can be many potential benefits for teens using social media. The US Surgeon General's 2023 Advisory (*Social Media and Youth Mental Health*) talks about the potential benefits for some youth, stating that social media can provide "positive community and connection with others who share identities, abilities, and interests." It can also provide "access to important information and create a space for self-expression," while online relationships and friendships can "afford opportunities to have positive interactions with more diverse peer groups than are available to them offline and can provide important social support." Lastly, the report explains that "the buffering effects against stress that online social support from peers may provide can be especially important for youth who are often marginalized, including racial, ethnic, and sexual and gender minorities."[1]

Pre-pandemic, there were 2 billion social media users in the world that checked their social media platforms 150 times a day.[2] In the fall of 2019, just as my first book was released, I was invited to speak on Colorado Public Radio for the series "Teens Under Stress." At that time, researchers found that in the previous two years, the national rate of teen anxiety, depression, and death by suicide had increased some 60 percent.[3] The main contributors to this steep increase were higher academic stress and growing social media usage.

Then the pandemic hit. Children and teens were out of school and locked down at home. While males flocked to electronic gaming with their buddies, females tended to retreat to the isolation of their bedrooms and spent countless hours on social media apps.

During the deep days of COVID, we had to use Zoom and other communication platforms on our electronic devices to be in touch with family and friends. On the positive side, these apps helped our deep desire to connect with friends and find some needed entertainment, and in retrospect, social media and gaming were lifesavers throughout COVID.

At the same time, all this online activity left our children more isolated and more vulnerable to the negative impacts of social media. A survey conducted by the Royal Society for Public Health (RSPH) asked fourteen- to twenty-four-year-olds in the UK how social media platforms impacted their health and well-being. The survey results found that Snapchat, Facebook, Twitter, and Instagram all led to increased feelings of depression, anxiety, poor body image, and loneliness.[4] And that doesn't even include all the negative statistics related to TikTok!

While statistics on child or teen mental health have skyrocketed, further research suggests that females have higher levels of anxiety and depression than males by 28 percent.[5] The theory as to why is often linked to how the two genders use their devices. Females tend to use social media apps for hours on end, alone in their rooms. These apps can create a plethora of self-comparison problems in all areas of a young person's life.

Young males, on the other hand, were busy electronic gaming with their friends. Wearing headsets, they could talk and laugh with each other, even though they were isolated in their own homes. Therefore, they didn't suffer the same level of social isolation compared with their female counterparts. In addition, a recent University of Colorado study, extremely reassuring for parents, did not find a connection between teen use of electronics and long-term adult life usage.[6]

In my own experience of working with young men after the lockdown, they reassessed their gaming habits around their junior year of high school. These past gamers now became engaged in driving, dating, extracurriculars, and were thinking about college. For young men with autism spectrum disorder (ASD), where social interaction is so overwhelming, I found that their COVID gaming obsessions continued into the late teens and early twenties.

The Brain on Social Media

Part of understanding what is happening in the brain begins with the dopamine system. **By design, social media also hijacks the desire,**

novelty, and reward system. Who can't resist watching another short video or that ding when we receive a new post? While hard to resist for adults, think about how that impacts the child and teen brain with an underdeveloped self-control center. It's hard to imagine that a lot of homework is getting done when those temptations are in the palm of their hands.

The rabbit hole of a hyper-focused time waste is made even worse because of the algorithms used by the apps. Based on your personal data and what you watch, or even just hover over for a couple seconds, the app serves more of what brings you pleasure and thus keeps you more engaged. As one teen male said to me in a lecture, "I keep getting reels of scantily clad girls!" I then described to him how the algorithms work as we had a laugh about what he was interested in.

Spiking Cortisol Levels

Negative experiences on social media can produce an increase in cortisol levels and a steady stream of stress. While a teen might be happy and excited when others like their posts, what about when they get a negative response to a post or even worse no response at all? Imagine the internal dialogue: "Why did she say that?" "Do others think the same thing?" "Why isn't anyone responding?" "I feel so invisible."

Research has found that females (males can also experience this) are particularly susceptible to comparing their bodies and appearance to other females.[7] Scrolling through a variety of perfect photos of other teen girls, it's hard to remember that each photo has been highly choreographed, edited, and airbrushed before it was posted. The self-talk then becomes: "I don't look nearly as nice." "I'm so fat compared to her." "I'll never look that good."

This type of negative self-talk and self-shaming can easily lead to what's called body dysmorphia, in which one can't see themselves accurately and never feels satisfied with how they look. Given all the pro-eating disorder sites and posts, you can see what's coming next.

We also cannot forget the well-known concept of FOMO (fear of missing out). Imagine how anyone might feel when they see posts from a social event or fabulous vacation that they are not experiencing in their lives. Will someone be happy that they weren't invited to the event as they'd rather just stay home? Will they think about the hassles of holiday travel? Probably not. A child, and especially teens, hate to feel left out of anything.

Can you recall a time when you experienced the visceral pain of not being invited to a birthday party? That internal dialogue sounds something like: "Why didn't I get invited?" "What's wrong with me?" "Why am I always left out?" "No one likes me."

As we will see in the next section, humans, by design, are quick to compare their lives to others. Even if your child might have been perfectly happy playing with their siblings at home over break, that can turn pretty negative when they see pictures of a friend on the beach in Mexico.

The Mirror Neuron System

A brief description of the mirror neuron system will help you understand why social media can be so damaging to your child's brain. Located in the right hemisphere, mirror neurons are essential to your child's social skills development and the source of empathy.

To understand how the mirror neuron system works, imagine that you are looking at a smile on your child's face. While not being conscious of it, your brain is now firing and stimulating the same muscles in your face that your child's face is using to smile. After stimulating those similar muscles, your brain then thinks: "If I was doing that, I'd feel happy. Therefore, my child is feeling happy." In other words, in a fraction of a second, we are constantly imitating what we observe so as to understand what others are thinking and feeling. With that knowledge, we can then hopefully formulate a socially appropriate and empathetic way to respond to others. What an amazing system.

When we text or use other messaging services, however, our communication lacks the nonverbal cues that activate our understanding of other people's emotions, which is our empathy system. Texts can hurt the receiver unintentionally. Without the emotional cues, it is easy to misinterpret what is being said. Negotiating the ups and downs of social relationships takes real time, in-person communication.

Given how the mirror neuron system works, humans can be influenced towards positive self-development and positive interactions as we live and work with others. At the same time, however, humans are amazingly vulnerable to negative influences.

Given that we are both a predator and prey species, our brains are wired to notice negative threats in the environment. News outlets have known forever that negative, threatening news sells papers and drives viewership. That's also true for things that are sensational and exciting. As my dad used to say, "Sex sells."

When it comes to social media, research has found that misinformation spreads six times faster than factual, credible information.[8] Why? It's more exciting and more titillating as it activates our mirror neurons. We might think: "If those people are worried about something, then I should be as well." "If those people are having a great time vaping or drinking alcohol or acting sexy, then I should be doing that too." "Look at all those kids having fun, and I wasn't even invited."

There are many old-fashioned phrases used by parents to describe our vulnerable system, such as: "Monkey see, monkey do." "If your friend jumped off a cliff, would you do it as well?" "Don't worry so much what your friends think." "Take your six best friends, and that will describe who you are."

In the research, we see this play out for those who are trying to stop smoking cigarettes. If you keep hanging out with friends who smoke, you will have a harder time quitting.[9] Our mirror system also explains why humans are so vulnerable to advertising and social media algorithms. In the classroom, every teacher knows that it takes only a couple of kids to look at each other and laugh before the laughter spreads like wildfire. We are, in fact, copycats.

These impacts on your child or teen can also be seen in the adult world on both a micro and macro level. In a March 2023 *Science Friday* podcast, journalist Ira Flatow asked, "Has social media fundamentally changed how we interact with the world? And how did big tech companies accumulate so much unchecked power along the way?"[10]

In the podcast, Flatow interviews *New York Times* reporter Max Fisher and explains how his book *The Chaos Machine: The Inside Story of How Social Media Rewired Our Minds and Our World* looks at "social media's early promises to build a more just and democratic society," and yet, "over the past several years, we've seen its propensity to easily spread hate speech, misinformation and disinformation."[11] Fisher's book also talks about how "online platforms have even played a role in organizing violent acts in the real world, like genocide against the Rohingya people in Myanmar, and the violent attempt to overturn the election at the United States capitol."[12]

Most interesting to me is how users feel a desire to post more rageful comments when they receive likes for their rageful posts. It seems as if these outcomes are knowingly "baked" into how these social media platforms are designed.[13]

The Teen Brain

Children are wired to make friends and connect with others. It is the essence of how we survive as a species. This is especially true for the teen brain. As a child, your family took care of you; as an adult, it is your peers who will take care of you. So, while things like appearance and social acceptance are important for children, these issues are paramount for teens. Unfortunately, social media delivers more content than the brain can keep up with or make sense of.

At puberty, massive changes take place that will help your teen learn to survive, work, and play with peers. As for the social brain areas discussed so far, I have developed a simple formula: **1/2 the frontal lobe + twice the emotional output + an explosion of the mirror neuron system = TEEN ANGST.**

For teens, the dopamine levels drop in half. This lack of impulse control and a tendency toward distractibility made teenagers more able to hear noises or see movement and then jump into action so as to protect the group. Today, lower dopamine levels make teens frequently feel bored.

Teenagers can get an instant dopamine boost when they post on social media or imitate the last TikTok challenge. Spurred by a flood of hormones, the doubling of emotional output makes them intense creatures who are quick to anger (useful in battle) and who are equally intense about bonding with others and seeking out romance. That expanded mirror neuron system is helping them become tomorrow's leaders, but also leads to a hyper-focused state about what others think and what others are doing.

The worst possible fear for a teen is to be embarrassed (usually by their parents) in front of their peers. Beneath it all is our most ancient fear: the fear of being rejected by the group. In ancient cultures if you were kicked out of the group, you would most likely die.

These changes in the teen brain also make them prone to extremely mean behavior as they jockey for social positions and try to fit in with the cool group by making fun of someone who's lower on the popularity scale. While that behavior has always occurred with teens, think about how teens can be even crueler with anonymous posts. With social media, a teen's fear of embarrassment is now broadcast far and wide with no way to delete it.

As a parent, think about your most embarrassing teen moment and how much more devastated you would have been if that moment had been on social media. Before social media, you could go home after school and get some sort of break from the day's embarrassments and frustrations. If phones are in the room, a 24/7 obsession keeps teens from developing the all-important skill of emotional compartmentalization. That means being able to box up your negative emotions and get on with the rest of your life.

As far as the impact of social media on teen females, it's important to understand that at puberty, the mirror neuron system becomes twice as dense in their brains compared to males. The process is sped up by estrogen, so this means that females notice much more than the average male and process the information twice as fast.[14] If social media is positive, they feel great. If it's negative input, they are devastated.

In regard to teens, Aristotle said it best: "Teens today are as fickle in their desires as they are vehement in expressing them." Or, as I like to tell my students, "If Romeo had just chilled out and waited, Juliet would have woken up."

While the teen brain takes years to develop, the average age for the onset of puberty in females has dropped from age 16.5 at the turn of the twentieth century to the current age of 12.5.[15] While cognitive development is going to take another decade or so, social media inundates the teen brain with endless streams of information about the adult world, which they are not emotionally ready to handle. It's one of the reasons why, in 2022, depressed and suicidal adolescents often spent days or weeks in exam rooms waiting for pediatric beds to open up.[16] Emergency rooms were simply overwhelmed.

That shattering statistic reflects the social and emotional brain, but also includes other issues like misinformation, overly negative news, the lack of "in real life" (IRL) social skills development, the explosion in pornography sites, sexting, sextortion, and the promotion of self-destructive behavior such as cutting, eating disorders, and suicide. This list gets longer everyday while our children's mental health continues to decline.

Shame-Free Parenting Tips to Help Manage Social Media

1. Embrace it.

While parent groups and governmental leaders are trying to rein in social media sites, they aren't going away. The positive side is how we are able to connect with our friends and families and even find some entertainment. There are also a host of positive support groups. We know from the research that a five- to ten-minute break to watch kitten and puppy videos can relax the brain and make us more productive.[17]

2. Be a role model.

The majority of American adults are now on social media apps. I have an Instagram account that I check a couple times a day for five minutes. If you don't want your child to get carried away, you have to demonstrate restraint as well. Next time you are ready to get upset with your child's usage, try and put some limits around your own usage. Create some phone free places and times for the whole family. Then remember to keep them out of sight and out of mind for everyone. You might want to check out a biometric storage box like Trova.[18]

3. Consider waiting on the smartphone.

Like most parents, we were considering letting our daughter have a smartphone when she was in sixth grade (that's when we saw other parents doing so). At the same time, we felt mixed because in our professional work we saw all the struggles that middle school children were having with social media.

Thankfully, we discovered the Wait Until 8th organization. Started by a mom, the organization provides support for parents who feel like they have to cave to the smartphone generation before their child is mature enough to handle the many temptations. We then decided to wait until the start of high school before giving her a phone. While she made a lot of noise about it at the time, she later thanked us because she saw how much trouble she had prevented in her life by not getting a phone sooner. As for me and my wife, we have never had a moment of thinking we should have given her one sooner. When it comes to social media, it's a huge Pandora's Box!

4. Find a motivating reason.

When discussing getting a smartphone with your child, start by talking about their motivators for having one, such as staying in touch with friends, not being left out of social opportunities, and the desire to learn more online.

Write those reasons down and talk about how those are things that are positive and will make them feel good. Then talk about how too much social media can make you feel bad about yourself. That becomes one of your gold standards for monitoring social media usage. If your child is feeling happy from it, great. If not, then it's time to trim back.

5. Start slow with freedoms of use.

Just like you set freedom-of-use rules for your teen driver and the car, smartphone usage requires the same protocol. Start with time limits on the phone and then take it away when that time is reached. Also have rules on using it in public spaces and not in the bedroom. In addition, have your teen turn off notifications when doing homework or spending time with the family.

Most important, phones must be turned in to the parents' bedroom every night for recharging. No excuses. You'll want to increase these freedoms as time goes by with responsible usage. After all, your child will be out of the house some day and will be better off if they learned how to manage things under your watch.

Part of your "freedoms of use" discussions should be about the various social media apps you are comfortable with. Then check your child's phone periodically to make sure these apps aren't being used. Many a parent has been horrified by seeing that their child's posts on social media or simple text threads are way out of control.

You can also research various parenting controls for the device or the internet service. To be honest, I haven't found many of these that teens can't find a way to work around.

6. Discuss when to seek out adult support.

Once your child is on social media, participates in group gaming, or even just looks at YouTube videos, you need to talk to them about the many things to look out for: cyber-bullying, sexting (never send it, keep it, or forward it), cat fishing (predators pretending to be children), sextortion (predators getting children to send naked photos so they can hold them for ransom), pornography sites, and posts that promote self-harm (cutting, eating disorders, foolish pranks, or suicide) or threats to others' safety, including homicide.

You'll also need to talk to younger users about how even typing a common word in the search bar (maybe your child wants to learn about some type of beaver) might lead them to all sorts of other content.

Finally, discuss how, as a child or teen, they are not equipped to handle or stop a friend who is posting about suicide. Many times, I've thanked a teenager for contacting me about a friend who was making these kinds of posts. You'll also want to talk about blocking someone who is bullying them. As I told one fifth grader, "If it makes you feel bad about yourself, block that person or site."

7. Use media resources.

Talk to your children about how social media works. Explain algorithms and how these companies make money. You can also talk about how these companies want to attract younger users so they will become life-long users. A good film to watch together is *Social Dilemma*, which contains lots of clips of children and teens talking about their experiences.

For a broader reach, encourage your child's school to sign up with the Social Institute. Started by Laura Tierney, the Institute produces videos (including those co-created by teens) on how to keep social media usage positive. If you go to my podcast, *Legit Parenting*, you can listen to my interview with Laura.[19]

Also, explore sites and posts created by teens who recognize the problems with social media and who are trying to make a positive contribution to teen mental health. Here are a couple to check out: Instagram's JackStrong17, created by a group of young men whose friend died by suicide; and Mary Walker's Instagram called "a.little. love.and.smiles".[20] In another words, you can find flowers in any barren wasteland.

8. Discuss Artificial Intelligence (AI).

When I first began working on my podcast and this book, AI was still a vision of the future. We don't yet know what the future of AI will look like for our kids and grandchildren, and while AI holds some amazing promises, it also has its perils. Start by talking to your children about academic integrity and about how using AI to write your paper is cheating. Then let them know what the consequence will be if they are caught doing so.

In the spring of 2023, a few teens told me about getting Chat GPT. Early on, I asked one of them, a high achiever who started college at the age of sixteen and loves all the learning he does digitally, to explain it to me as we were playing the card game Uno. He spontaneously asked the program to describe the statistical probabilities related to winning the card game. Within seconds, it typed out a six-page document. I've never seen anything like it.

As AI proliferated, it wasn't too long before I started hearing from more teens about how they use the program to write their school papers. (I remember using CliffsNotes for various books I read in school, but I still had to type the paper.) I asked about teachers who scanned papers back into AI to see if they were AI produced. The answer to that was: "You just rewrite parts of your paper so you don't get caught!"

As with all the other apps discussed already, take a periodic look at your children's AI app to see what it's being used for. You can also scan one of their papers back into Chat GPT to find out if the program generated it. Finally, from what I've been reading and listening to, Chat GPT is not always accurate. That would also be a good thing to let your children and teens know.

CHAPTER 6

VALIDATING EMOTIONS: GUNS, SCHOOL SHOOTINGS, AND OTHER IMMEDIATE STRESSORS

In this chapter, we will begin exploring how to validate your child's emotions, especially when something upsetting happens unexpectedly in their life and creates an immediate stressor.

With traumatic events, as parents, you experience your own stress and need to decide if and when you should discuss that stressor with your children. Examples of these situations could be the death of an animal or family member, a cancer diagnosis in the family, or a mass shooting of some sort. Situations of immediate trauma will shake you to your core and challenge your parental abilities.

These types of situations precipitate numerous calls to my office. Helping your child develop insight into how they feel and how to express their emotions appropriately is a skill that will benefit them throughout their life. Draining off your child's excess emotions, like releasing flood gates when the dam is about to overflow, can also prevent negative expressions and stress-induced behavioral problems.

Should I Bring Up the Situation?

Sadly, our children are experiencing school shootings (and other mass shootings) at an alarming rate. There were forty-six school shootings in 2022, and 2023 appeared to be on a record pace.[1] Here in Denver, the premier school for Denver Public Schools, East High School, experienced two shootings only weeks apart in the spring of 2023. The first was when a student athlete was shot to death while sitting in his car in front of the school. The second occurred when a student shot two administrators and then later died by suicide.

As you watch or listen to news like this, parents are confronted with that difficult question: "Do I talk to my child right away or wait to see how the story unfolds?" This is tricky because you want to shelter your kids from some of life's bigger tragedies and the fears and anxieties that accompany them.

Preschoolers are still worried about monsters under their beds, getting used to school, and being separated from their parents. Third graders' standard fears include feeling safe when they are away from you, school exams, and robbers coming when they hear noises at night as they fall asleep. Fears of night noise is standard for this age because they do not fully understand the mathematical concept of statistical probability (i.e., how many homes might get broken into at night compared to how many homes went undisturbed).

As parents of teens, you worry that hearing about a suicide or school shooting might trigger some of these same thoughts in other teens or your own teen. At the same time, if you wonder whether or not you should talk to your child immediately about a traumatic event, know that your kids need to know about things in the world. You cannot wrap them in a bubble for their entire lives. That would be wrong because it hurts their development and their chances of becoming more resilient. We cannot bubble wrap our kids, but when is the appropriate time for them to learn about realities such as a mass shooting at a local grocery store?

As a parent, given the problems with playground rumors, I've always preferred talking about the "facts of life" directly to my kids versus them hearing it from other students. This is true for trauma situations but also for talking to my kids about the birds and the bees. I believe the best sex education begins at home, not on pornographic websites or social media platforms.

Assess Size and Closeness

One of your first considerations in deciding whether or not you want to talk about a traumatic event with your kids is: How big of an event is it? Consider how much coverage it's going to get and how close it is to the reality of your family life. In 1999, when the shooting at Columbine High School happened in Littleton, Colorado, it was on all the TV and news stations. I was on my way to my office, which was in a church a mile down the street from the school, listening to the coverage in my car.

Everybody in the community knew about it. There was no way you could not; there were so many helicopters flying overhead, sirens, and students running through neighborhoods for safety. All of the district schools were on lockdown. Everyone in the district knew something was going on and news of the event quickly spread to the Denver metro community and around the world in a matter of days (and that was before social media). In that situation, you had to talk to your children if you lived in the metro area of Denver. For families in other states and countries, you had a day or so to think about it.

On the morning of 9/11, the terrorist attack was taking place right as kids were going to school and almost the entire school had heard about it and was in a state of shock. I went around to the classrooms from kindergarten on up through eighth grade to talk to the children and help them process what was happening.

One of the most meaningful memories of my life was with an angelic first-grade girl. I had explained how many police officers and firefighters were injured as they tried to rescue people. Sweet Emily raised her hand and asked, "Mr. Knippenberg, why would anybody want to hurt firefighters or police officers? They're our heroes." As I choked up, all I could say at that moment was, "I don't know, honey. I can't answer that question." Sadly, there are going to be situations in your own parenting journey in which you're not going to know how to answer. **It's okay to tell your child, "I do not know."**

Some traumas might be contained to a smaller group of students, such as a specific class or grade level. We had a first-grade student who lost his mother suddenly to a heart attack several years back. All the first graders knew about it. I went to talk to the first graders right away, and then, given that the boy had friends in second grade, I also covered that grade level. Putting it all together, you have to think about how big the event is and how close it is to your family, school, or the community groups involved.

Your Own Emotions

As parents, you also need to consider your own emotional state prior to your children coming home. Children observe their parents' emotions; therefore parents should explain their emotions to their children in an age-appropriate manner. In doing so, you'll want to have some composure over your emotions and more adult/parental thoughts about the event, so you can tune in to how a child thinks and feels. You also need to prepare yourself in the event that your child expresses gut-wrenching emotions. These are "ugly" cries and take parental composure to validate their emotional experiences.

One of my first vivid memories is when I was about five. My mom was standing in front of the black-and-white TV set watching Walter Cronkite as he announced the assassination of President Kennedy. I didn't really understand who the President was, but I knew that a man had done a bad thing. What I really knew, and remember to this day, is that my mom was upset and that is what bothered me the most.

If you feel pretty overwhelmed, you may decide not to talk to your child right after school. It might be a good idea to get your ducks in a row first by talking with someone such as another parent, friends, or extended family members. Later in the evening is just fine, but you might want to turn off the TV or social media so your kids do not become aware of the situation before you are ready to talk. If that happens, simply say, "That's a really hard thing isn't it. I was planning on us having a family discussion later this evening after we know a little more information. We can talk about it now if you want to."

For myself, I visited with one of my former students who was locked down during the second 2023 shooting at East High School. He told me how he was locked in a dark room with no windows and watched his friends' video feeds of a body being taken out to an ambulance. Then, he looked at me and said, "I wasn't afraid for myself but for my friends who were on the first level of the school." I was so proud of this young man I've known since kindergarten but saddened that he and his classmates had to experience such a trauma. Obviously, I had to compose myself before meeting with my next appointment.

Consider Age

Before you talk to your child, you may also want to consider: Is this the time in your child's normal development to learn about a traumatic event or should you wait on this one? You, as the parent, have to decide if you tell your child thirty minutes from now or wait and see what they have heard about it. If you don't tell them, there may be a chance that tomorrow, on the playground, they will hear about it from some kids whose parents did talk to them. Or what are the chances a classmate who has older siblings or owns a smartphone tells their friends at school? After all, what child does not enjoy hearing some juicy bit of news and then lording it over their classmates?

So now the question is: Do you want your child to hear about it from you or from some kids? If you remember the game Telephone, then you know how inaccurate communication between classmates can be. The so-called facts they hear from other kids are often confused or completely wrong and often sensationalized.

Never underestimate what kids hear at school. They hear all sorts of stuff. News trickles down fast. If your child has classmates with older siblings, then they are probably going to hear about traumatic events that are happening in the world.

Sixth to Twelfth Graders

If you have a sixth to twelfth grader and the event is reasonably large and there is a good chance it will be discussed by students or teachers (we do want older students to think critically about events in the world), I'd say talk to them that evening for sure. Many of their classmates are going to have older siblings, and smartphones have become a standard issue for teens. Even if you are waiting until high school for your child to have a smartphone, plenty of their classmates will have them.

Fifth Graders

Think about how almost every elementary school day starts. It usually begins with a morning check-in for fourth and fifth graders. During these morning activities, you need to remember that one or two kids might say something about the event.

Developmentally, fifth graders want to feel more independent from you. They want to feel like they are older, that they can ride their bikes to the mall or the grocery store and be with their friends at the park. They do not want to have playdates anymore; they just want to go play without adult supervision.

But here's the risk with fifth graders: You might be able to get away without telling them, and maybe they won't hear about it the next day. However, many of their friends will have heard about it when they come to school the next day. If you do not talk to them, you run the risk of them being really upset with you, believing you do not trust them, that you do not think they are old enough to know about events, and that you are trying to hide things from them. This will be their natural response.

Third to Fourth Graders

Third to fourth graders are the trickiest age for deciding when to talk to them about large traumatic events. If there has been a history of some of the kids in the third and fourth grade telling all the other kids about stuff they are hearing from their teenage brothers and sisters, then you might want to have a conversation. If not, you can see how it goes in the afternoon or early evening and see if your child brings it up.

You can also go with a simple and subtle query like: "How was school today? What were you kids talking about on the playground? Any announcements from your teacher?" It's like fly fishing. You throw out some lines and see if you get any bites. If you do, then you can decide to talk more about the event.

What is difficult about talking with younger children is that they are naturally starting to understand the realities of the world at the same time they are starting to understand statistical probability. If a younger child thinks that this bad thing is happening everywhere and happens all the time, then they will have a lot more anxiety. (See chapter 7 for ways to help your child with statistical probability.)

Kindergarten to Second Graders

For kindergarten to second grade, you probably don't want to talk to them about the traumatic event unless it's really close to them in their lives or is something from their direct circle of classmates or friends.

At our school, I will swing by the front door of these classrooms and just greet the younger classes from the door. If the teacher says, "Hi Mr. Knippenberg, why don't you come in?" it means that the kids have been talking about the event, and I need to come and address the class. If the teacher just gives me a nod, it means that they are all good.

Following the shooting at East High School in the spring of 2022, a first-grade teacher met me in the hall with two students. She asked me to chat privately with just them. We sat outside, and I processed their emotions from the event the day before. It was so sweet when they said: "Our parents told us about it but told us not to tell the other students, so we haven't." What a relief.

At the same time, younger children pick up bits of information from peers and then create a variety of scenarios in their minds. In the spring of 2022, a parent emailed me about a disturbing chat she had with her second-grade daughter. Thankfully, this student opened up to her mother about her worries of some man running around schools and shooting children. She then said that she heard that if you were in a bathroom during such an event, you wouldn't be able to run to the classroom. She then asked her mom, "What do I do if my teacher is shot?" The mother emailed me, saying, "This conversation cut me to the bone. I didn't know what to say." I assured the second grader when I met with her about proper protocol that there wasn't someone running loose that was coming to her school. I was then able to find out who she heard this from and talked to those students as well. Sadly, it's true that "Little pitchers have big ears."

What's even more difficult is the new security systems that are being implemented in schools around the country. While we expect younger ones to accept the new "locked doors" policy, and electronic pass cards on lanyards for older students, they often figure out the fear behind it and then anticipate an impending attack. It's no different than my experience of hiding under my desk for the imminent nuclear attack. Even in third grade, I knew that my little desk wouldn't save me.

Preschoolers

For preschoolers, I generally do not discuss big events with the whole class unless there is a direct impact on all the students. During COVID, in the fall of 2020, we had several preschool children who were showing regressive signs, such as soiling their pants and being extra needy. I did a whole class talk on wearing masks and not being close to each other and then helped them learn about how living through stressful times can make us behave like we were younger.

Shame-Free Parenting Tips for Talking to Your Kids About Stressful Things

1. Know how your child processes emotions.

Children have their own natural temperaments and ways of processing emotions. A temperament is the one or two emotions that seem to come out more under stress. It could be that a child defaults to anxiety when they hear about difficult things. Other children might become sad or more depressed. Another reaction could be anger. When discussing the shooting at the King Soopers in Boulder, Colorado, in the spring of 2021, I had one middle school student express a great deal of anger over our country's gun control policy.

Some children might not want to talk on an emotional level, while another child might immediately think about how to make others feel better. All of these reactions are just fine.

In terms of actually talking about the events, you might have a child who wants to process the events with you and explore a variety of details and emotions. You might also have a child who is a bit of a stoic. They might want to process it more internally and focus on how to move forward versus focusing on the emotional pain.

If your child does not seem to be impacted by the event, then do not make it a bigger deal than they think it is (even though, as a parent, you feel shaken to your core). You can always circle back to it later to see how they are dealing with it.

2. Center yourself.

Some ways you can help your child feel open to talking about traumatic events is to have a snack with them or do something together like working with your hands. Teens might do better talking about events while you are driving (although they'll need to take their ear buds out) or talking at the family dinner table while you eat.

You can say something like: "I/we need to talk to you about something upsetting that happened today" or "Did you hear about what happened today?"

3. Lay out the ground rules.

You can set the ground rules for your family and say, "Whatever feelings or thoughts you have about what we are talking about is okay. Everyone reacts to difficult things in life in their own way. Say anything you want about it and ask any questions you want."

With siblings of different ages, remind them that we do not judge others' thoughts, questions, or feelings. The last thing a younger child needs is an older sibling who calls them stupid or laughs at them when they ask a question.

4. Stick to the facts you know.

When talking about a mass shooting, for younger children, you might start with a frame of reference that they can understand. One approach is to say, "You know how sometimes some of your classmates get upset and then hit another child? Well, sometimes older people get upset and react physically instead of using their words."

Another possible approach is to say, "Do you remember how your pet fish died unexpectedly? Well, that also happens with other animals and people."

For older children, you can jump in more quickly by saying, "Something really sad happened today. A person(s) went into ____ and started ____. They do not know yet why the person(s) did this. It sounds like numerous people were ____."

Stay calm when your child asks any follow up questions. Answer them simply: "They used a ____" or "The doctor/police said ____." It's also okay to say, "No one knows that yet." Stay away from gory details or information about what kinds of guns were used.

5. Validate emotions.

Next, direct the discussion to how your child feels about it. You can start with one of your basic feelings to get things started. The key here is to simply validate the emotion they feel. You can also simply explain the feeling of being in shock and how it might take a while for your child to know how they feel.

You might also agree to turn the TV off and ask your children to not pay attention to what's being said on social media or on the school playground. Encourage them not to listen to or spread rumors. Remind your child that they can come to you with any questions.

Remember, you do not have to do this all in one sitting. You can come back to it later that day or the next morning or afternoon.

6. Reinforce safety.

Younger ones will struggle with geographical proximity, that they have been to the place where the event happened, so they might feel that all areas are unsafe. Reassure them that they are safe right now and that it's your job to keep them as safe as possible. Then explain that the schools do fire/lockdown drills for safety reasons.

You might also want to talk about what to do at home when a tornado alarm goes off, or there is smoke, or the smell of egg in the house. While these drills might produce anxiety for some children, it is better than not knowing what to do in a situation. A survivor in the East High School shooting talked about how he remembered his school drills and knew what to do.

For in-the-moment emergencies, your child might not know what to do. This was exemplified by a mother in Florida who was trapped upstairs with flood waters rising, saying to her daughter, "Stop crying. I need you to have your wits about you. There will be time for tears tomorrow."

For a little insight, ask your children if they can think of one game that children around the world play: Hide and Seek. It's a way for children to learn how to run and hide to protect themselves from danger.

You can also remind them that a child's scream is the world's first alarm system. In the event of something happening at school, you can tell them that statistically, schools report far less injuries to children than any other place.[2] Lots of rules and adult eyes keep kids safe.

7. Plan to do something.

One of the most amazing things my son and I did the afternoon of 9/11 was to go to Berry Patch Farms in Brighton, Colorado, where you pick your own berries. We just sat and worked with our hands, picking raspberries, and eating a few as we worked. It was incredibly grounding.

The next afternoon, we baked a cake with his friend and used the raspberries and some blueberries to make an American flag on top of the white icing. We took it to the firehouse just down the street from our school and thanked the firefighters. That was a great thing.

Talk to your kids about what you can do. After the 2018 Parkland, Florida, school shooting, my daughter placed roses and a handmade poster for each student who was lost on the altar at her school. You can also donate money to those who are in need. Perhaps you can find a GoFundMe sight for victims' families and the traumatized survivors. The important part is to help your family turn your empathy into a verb.

8. Dig deeper into larger social issues.

For older children, this is an excellent time to look at issues surrounding the event in a deeper way and then look at opportunities for civic action.

Tragically, one in four teens reported they could get a loaded gun in twenty-four hours. **Half of those teens said they could do so in**

less than ten minutes.[3] How twisted is that for our children? Your teen could get involved in promoting increased mental health services in schools, or perhaps they will want to get involved in sensible gun legislation and be active in organizing gun violence protests just like the students in Florida have done.[4] After the Columbine shooting, I took my young son down to a protest in favor of sensible gun legislation.

Adding to the problem are online interactions that result in drive-by shootings or shooting up birthday parties. The Black community has been particularly affected with the glorification of the gun culture. Sadly, one famous basketball player recently was photographed twice brandishing a gun. Is that really a role model for peace, acceptance, and success? NBA Commissioner Adam Silver placed a twenty-five-game suspension on Ja Morant, stating, "The potential for other young people to emulate Ja's conduct is particularly concerning."[5]

One thing that came from the Black Lives Matter (BLM) movement is awareness of systematic forms of oppression, or even systematic racism. This is where groups of people are suffering because of written or unwritten rules that keep them from having a fair chance or a level playing field.

When I was a kid, BIPOC (Black, indigenous, and people of color) populations lived in their own neighborhoods; they weren't allowed in white neighborhoods. It was very segregated. While the Fair Housing Act stopped formal rules of segregation, it unfortunately didn't mean that BIPOC populations could get home loans. Even today, BIPOC communities have less home equity to pass on to future generations because they're discriminated against for getting home loans. That's a systemic issue. You can talk to your kids about systemic oppression. You can join a protest. We had a number of students at our school who joined in BLM protests.

As you are looking at civic activities for your kids, have them study a little history. They could learn about why the Alamo took place or how the play *Hamilton* shows that slavery was kept in our constitution so that the northern and southern states could be united. You could even look at reconstruction after the Civil War and the passing of Jim Crow laws. There is so much to delve into and then have deep conversations about it with your older children.

9. Look for emotions in play.

As time goes by from your first conversation, you'll want to observe your child's play activities to gauge how they are feeling. Kids display their thoughts and emotions in their play because play is how younger kids figure out the world.

Perhaps you had a nice family discussion with them about a traumatic event, but don't be surprised if later that day or the next day you hear that they were on the school playground imitating what happened. The day after the Columbine shooting, we had young elementary students playing gun games. The adults were horrified, but that's how kids process things.

After 9/11, we had a couple of kids pretending to be airplanes crashing into the playground structures. As an adult, your reaction might be, "Oh my God, that's just horrendous!" Rather than being upset, however, you have to appreciate what is going on and take the time to say in a calm voice, "Let's talk about what you were playing." Then you can talk about how confusing and upsetting the particular event was and that it is normal to play it out in order to feel some control over it.

Then you might want to say, "Playing like this might be upsetting to others, so how about we play other games? We can talk about that event any time you want."

10. Foster hope.

When dealing with violence and tragic events such as shootings and mass murder, I remind my students that the world is much safer now than it's ever been. Back in the day, it's estimated that up to 40 percent of people worldwide died a violent death. Today it's less than 1 percent.[6] That's a very small fraction compared to the number of people in the past.

At the same time, 1 percent of people dying a violent death is still too many. This is the same with other tragic events, such as death from a cancer diagnosis or death from a car accident.

Throughout the talking process, help your kids develop a sense of hope. Talk to them about how they are safe and how they can make a difference. We want to keep building up hope for the future. One of my favorite lines by the philosopher Friedrich Nietzsche is: "Out of chaos comes a dancing star." I share this with students and remind them that we want to be that dancing star.

CHAPTER 7

VALIDATING EMOTIONS: LONG-TERM STRESS

While many of the strategies from chapter 6 on immediate stress and trauma will apply to the scenarios discussed in this chapter, there are some unique features about long-term stress and trauma that require additional strategies. These long-term stressors might be caring for a family member with cancer, meeting the needs of a medically challenged child, raising a child with a severe mental illness, long-term job loss, chronic food or housing insecurity, caring for a family member with dementia, a nasty divorce that continues on for years, or trying to survive day-to-day life throughout a pandemic.

My earliest memory of such a chronic stressor was at the age of eleven, when my parents decided to bring home my aging grandfather who was struggling with dementia (called hardening of the arteries back then). The brunt of the workload was on my mother as she endured countless bouts of Grandpa Knipp's confusion followed by anger and rage. While I tried to help out, I watched my mom's nerves frazzle away. The stress was simply too much. After what seemed like years, my father agreed that it was time for a nursing home.

The Toll of Chronic Stress

In April of 2021, I read a poignant article in the *Wall Street Journal* entitled "The Pandemic's Terrible Toll on Kids." It begins with a teen female who says, "I don't know how to feel, all the people I look up to, they're all like breaking down." She grew anxious about going to school, afraid she would catch the virus and spread it to her parents. (That's a huge fear for so many kids and teens who knew that it wasn't that dangerous for them but knew it could be deadly for older adults and those who had compromised immune systems.) Making matters worse, she talked about classmates who didn't believe in COVID and would purposely pull their masks down or not wear them in the hallways. Finally, she discussed the ongoing monotony and fatigue of chronic stress: "Every day is the exact same. You feel like what's the point."[1]

For this, I like to use the analogy of being on a long vacation or break. After a week or so, you begin to lose track of the days of the week. It's such a great feeling when you have made the choice to take time off and relax. It's not so great when it's caused by a pandemic or another similar situation. There is so much you want to do, but you can't. It's like being stuck in quicksand. If you fight it, your emotional health will sink lower. You just must relax and accept it while you look for a branch or two to stabilize your sinking mood.

In the research, countless children and teens experienced social isolation during the lockdown, and it was particularly hard on teens and college students who had to return home.[2] At this stage of development, their brains are wired to be connecting with peers and asking them not to is a Herculean task. Family stress skyrocketed with chronic worries about the virus, disruptions in family routines, school closures, remote learning, economic recession, and job loss. The list went on and on.

Even worse is the fact that children pick up on their parent's anxiety and stress, which makes them even more stressed and anxious. Research is also finding that all the family time under stress caused a rise in child abuse, neglect, parental substance abuse, parental depression and anxiety, and suicide.[3] After a year and a half of the pandemic, newly opening court rooms saw a surge in divorce filings.

While family togetherness can have some positives, it's pretty clear that we weren't meant to have this much family time together. Ancient families spent their days hunting, gathering, and working in the fields. They were not sitting together in the house all day.

The big question is: What's going to be the long-term effect from all of this? We are seeing a massive growth in children and teens who are experiencing anxiety and depression. In 2022, of all the concerns parents had for their children, struggling with anxiety or depression was at the top of the list with 76 percent of parents reporting that they were "somewhat" and "very" concerned for their child's mental health.[4]

We also know that children and adults with pre-existing traumas or mental health conditions will suffer the most. Those who have experienced what's called adverse childhood experiences (past traumas of various sorts) can have physical responses to stress that can damage the brain and immune system. This results in health issues such as depression, diabetes, obesity, cancer, cardiovascular disease, and substance abuse.[5]

Cortisol Comes to Town

Even without past traumas, we know that the amygdala (the fight, flight, or freeze area of the brain) releases cortisol. As discussed in the chapters on electronic gaming and social media, the amygdala's release of cortisol plays an important role in our survival when faced with immediate life or death situations. Those cortisol spikes are essential, but we want the levels to drop back down fairly quickly.

When cortisol levels stay elevated (maybe slightly lower than the high spikes seen in emergencies) you see some of the symptoms listed above. You can also see this cortisol impact on our faces. Skin needs oil, water, and the microbiome to be healthy and protective. Cortisol depletes all three. If you have noticed some recent aging lines, that's probably why. During the pandemic, teens and adults also saw an increase in acne from stress and from having to wear masks throughout the day.

Cortisol has an impact on our executive functioning system (the President) and our memory. Compared to stresses like 9/11 or hurricanes, where we can get on with the work of rebuilding, cortisol levels can come back down relatively quickly compared with chronic levels.

Academic scores among fourth and eighth graders took a big hit as well in 2022. Nationally, the average math score for fourth graders fell five points since 2019, while the average score for eighth graders dropped eight points (the biggest drop ever recorded). Average scores in reading for both grades fell three points.[6]

We've also looked at the allure of video games and social media and how these, too, increase cortisol levels on their own. Gaming and TikTok is winning out over homework, resulting in even poorer academic performance. Isolation and electronics have been the perfect storm for decreasing cognitive development. Even before the pandemic, anxiety, depression, and suicide rates among teens had reached record levels in 2019. Although the spring of 2020 showed some decreases in these trends as students faced less academic stress and were surrounded by family, those numbers bounced back to epidemic proportions during the spring of 2021. It is clear that the 2019 conditions were exasperated by this long period of stress.[7]

Decreasing Stress and Cortisol

Fortunately, we have learned plenty about how to protect ourselves and our children from these statistics. A study in the greater Seattle area found that the children and teens who were doing the best are the ones who have structured routines. The study also found that students who got more exercise and had less screen time had fewer behavior problems, less anxiety, and less depression.[8] As we will look at in the next chapter, students who have maintained a sense of purpose, and a set of goals related to that purpose, have been more resilient to chronic stress.

In our own home, our daughter held up pretty well emotionally in the spring of 2020. While online school was not a positive experience for any of us, she did finish her eighth-grade year. The summer of 2020 went well with our structured family life, with normal bed and wake times, and with her diving into all sorts of hobbies, but she was longing for high school and a new set of friends.

Her freshman year had lots of online learning at first and then just a few mornings a week later on. As the holidays came and went, we saw a big dip in her enthusiasm and motivation while her irritability largely increased. The spring of 2021 became increasingly difficult as we were all tired of so much time together, and she longed for in-person friendships. Thankfully, she turned sixteen over the summer, started driving, and got a job at a local fast food restaurant. The access to kids her own age miraculously changed her life and mental health.

When she started back to in-person school in the fall of 2021, that also made a huge difference. She didn't care about wearing a mask at school because she was with real friends, which was something her smartphone couldn't give her the year before.

As the fall of 2022 approached, we were dealing with the same normal problems that parents of teens have: never seeing her, concerns about her grades, and her spending too much time with friends. While these problems are still difficult for parents to deal with, we couldn't be happier!

Family Meetings

Changing emotional phases over long periods of time requires that you talk with your children. For starters, look for moments when your child, either through their words or through their behavior, is showing stress. Look especially for unexpected meltdowns. If you have had a child go through puberty, then you know how teenage emotions can change on a dime. They are fine one minute and then raging the next, coming out of nowhere like a thief in the night. The next minute they are happy again and you are left wondering what alien has possessed them. The same thing happens with any type of long-term stress. The stress can come out over the smallest, most random thing. When these moments happen, you have a direct window to their soul. You really want to just be aware and not overreact. Just be a mirror and say, "You're really struggling right now, aren't you? It's really hard. I know it's a hard time right now."

In addition to addressing these natural, emotion-filled moments, I strongly recommend regular, structured family meetings for chronic stress. These meetings, by the way, are also great for normal family life, especially with teens. Family meetings will also help your child learn to have more control over that window to their soul.

If you can, set a time for family meetings once a week. These could be on a weekend at a time that generally seems to work well for everyone's schedule. If you have younger children, it is important to avoid meeting later at night because the discussion could open up a lot of emotions around bedtime. As we all know, the brain is not very logical when it's tired. Opening the window to their soul at the point of fatigue means that the logical President has shut down, which can make the emotions even harder to turn off.

Many families find that after dinner is an effective time for serious discussions. Your main goal at this time is just to drain off emotions and then make any necessary adjustments to your family plan. You can ask questions, such as, "How are we doing as a family?" "What are our positives?" "Do we have some growth areas?" "What can we do to take care of these issues?"

Just talking about what things are like can do so much. When dealing with something like cancer, you can talk about how everyone is doing with dad being gone most nights to be at the hospital with a grandparent or how mom or dad will be more tired next week after chemo.

All Emotions Are Okay

The main rule here is that all our emotions are okay. And we do not want to judge anybody, especially the siblings. As a parent, you might just offer up the chance to talk about how everyone is feeling, or you could have a structured format.

For middle and high school students, I love to start with, "Does anybody have a joy, a success, a worry, or a sorrow that they'd like to share?" I am offering them a framework.

Some families with younger kids will do something less formal, like asking, "Who wants to share two or three roses from your day and one thorn?" I had one girl tell me that she was feeling like a sandwich.

When I queried further, she said, "I'm a sandwich of mad and sad that's smooshed together." What a lovely description.

Having a question of the day helps children deal with loss and change. Dealing with loss of any kind is difficult. There can be periods of long-term stress impacting you as a parent. When this is the case, children naturally tend to see themselves as part of the cause of your stress. Obviously, this will cause a great deal of anxiety for them. Take some time to explain why other people, situations, or whatever abounds is causing stress in your life. Then explain how stress might be causing a teacher to be a little crabbier or causing you to be a little short-tempered, and while a parent or teacher might have put up with their silliness or shenanigans in the past, they aren't putting up with it now because of stress factors.

As you talk, you can break issues into categories. Some will fall under the category of things that we can't control and just have to accept and get used to. For example, your child might not have liked wearing a mask in school, but they had to accept the school's new rules during COVID. The other category can be things that we can have control over. For instance, we might be able to change the texture of the mask or change the nature of the straps.

For a problem like siblings going into each other's room all the time, you might decide it is time for bedroom locks on the door. I grew up in a family with five siblings, and I strongly believe in the concept. When our children are sad or upset, it is natural to want to help them get rid of those feelings. It is an ugly cry when you hear your child experiencing emotional pain. You might want to drain the emotion or brainstorm ways to make life better. For many, adopting an animal is a great solution to unmet emotional needs.

While the above strategies can help reduce some of these emotions, there will be times when you just need to let your child feel what they feel. It is not our job as parents to make them feel happy all the time, nor would that be good for them. My daughter once said to me: "Dad, stop trying to make me feel better."

If you reach this point with your child, it might be good to simply say, "You know, I'd probably feel the same way." Then disengage.

Accepting Ambiguity

Another thing to emphasize is that in stressful times, we have to accept ambiguity. Ambiguity means we do not know for sure what might happen. We might hope that this or that will happen, but we do not know for sure. Explain to your child that you might have to make a change and go with plan B or C or D or E or even F. Help your children temper their expectations and understand that while it is human nature to seek control when we are anxious, we cannot control all.

It is much more stressful when we do not know if something worse is going to happen or not. In one study, when told to brace for a shock, one group of test subjects was able to mobilize their physical and emotional resources to prepare, as they were sure the shocking event was going to happen. The subjects who were told they "might" get a shock could not prepare and in the end produced more stress than the other group.[9]

Stress that builds and builds in our lives is like an old Alfred Hitchcock film. He was a master of suspense. In his films, we're in the room and see the door; then we hear something outside the door. It's slowly opening and we're just terrified because we don't know what is outside coming in. Once the door is open, we see it and make an action plan.

Long-term stress is like being stuck in a movie where the door is slowly opening, and we do not know what is on the other side or when the other shoe is going to drop. When you plan with your children and they get their hopes up, be sure to talk about how no one can control things and that changes might happen that you didn't expect. Then have a contingency plan or two.

Shame-Free Parenting Tips to Deal With Long-Term Stress

1. Reinforce your family rules and structure.

As your problem-solving and contingency planning unfolds, make sure you remind your children about your rules and standards. For instance, let's say you were talking with your child about attending a birthday party during COVID and that the hosting parents had set a standard for social distancing. You want to make sure that your child understands your expectations that they comply, even though all the kids are from the same cohort at school.

Before they leave, go over your rules and guidelines. Talk about what temptations might arise and how they should handle those. Remind them to think about, "What would mom or dad say about this?" Like a young teen driver heading out to a party, it's good to go over the marching orders.

2. Track your emotions.

You can also consider writing down your family's rules and emotions. One family had a jar for losses and a jar for hopes. They would talk about and write down these emotions on a slip of paper and drop them in. For our family, we started a gratitude jar. Every night at dinner, we'd write on slips of paper a gratitude that each of us had from the day and drop them into the colorful jar our daughter designed. We also put the date on it. On New Year's Day, we dumped them out and read them. Mine got the biggest laugh from the day the shelter in place started. I wrote: "I'm happy to have two weeks off!" Who knew it would go on for so much longer.

You have to be intentional with your positive mindset activities because negative thoughts and feelings travel twice as fast in the brain as do positive ones. Personally, I find great strength in counting my blessings; however, that has taken years of practice.

3. Paint a picture.

You want to try and help your children understand life and what is going on for them. Then help them paint a picture in their mind of what is going on. Talk about how, while you cannot change a worldwide pandemic or other stressors that are out of your control, you can think about things that might help everyone feel a little back to normal.

For our granddaughter, getting to play with some Barbies with Grandma before going to school made all the difference. For me, simply getting to watch the annual Tour de France painted a picture of the greater world and made everything feel more normal to me. The same was true with watching college football.

For many, the simple joy of wandering down the aisles of a favorite store helped them to feel normal again. If you talk to your kids, you will find that a big-change event might be something really small that sets them back on track to feeling good again.

4. Fill your child's emotional cup.

The concept of filling a child's emotional cup has been around for decades. During chronic stress, children will tend to have their cups tip over and drain out much more easily. Pick something specific to notice in your children. In the classroom, a teacher might focus on acts of kindness. At home, it could be cooperating more around the house with chores or getting along better with one's siblings (this was a major source of stress for families during lockdown).

While I was having the chronic struggle of dyslexia as a child, I would retreat into the womb of our basement to try and read my book. My mother would bring down her homemade chocolate cookies for me. While they did not help me read, they made all the difference.

Another way to fill your child's emotional cup is to create nicknames. A Hungarian proverb reminds us that having a nickname communicates closeness, value, and love: *A child with many names is well loved.* One of my daughters is Shrimpy, and my son and I are Mack and Bob (a story for another day). At school, I love June Bug for one of my younger students.

Remember, you don't need over-the-top, unwarranted "you are more special than anyone" praise or ribbons for everything to fill your child's emotional cup. I am not big into that. Just focus on those small moments when you can say, "You are loved" and "I am so happy to be sharing time with you during these difficult circumstances."

5. Give positive reinforcement.

Look for ways to give positive messages to your child. One idea is to set up a jar that gets filled with a little craft store fuzzy every time something good and helpful is completed.

Years ago, researchers wanted to know how much time you should use positive reinforcement versus negative reinforcement if you wished to motivate a child to actually want to change their behavior. The answer: 80 percent positive and 20 percent negative.[10] These statistics came from a study of fifth grade boys who had ADHD, or in other words children who have lots of impulses and little self-control.

It is much easier to use positive reinforcement to shape behavior and build closeness with your kids in good times, and especially during rough times when they need extra positive emotions. These positive messages should be for doing as well as for being. You might compliment a student for raising their hand or waiting their turn in line. Later, it might be letting your child know how much you appreciate and care about them.

6. Explain loss.

I like to think of life as a constant collection of pieces of glass. We are making sense of our life every day by collecting the pieces and then putting them together into a stained-glass window. This process helps us make sense out of our lives.

Sometimes, a small thing might happen that scuffs a piece of glass. For example, maybe your child's friend doesn't want to be friends anymore. Parents and teachers might try to patch the empty feeling by helping them realize that there are other friends to hang out with.

Parents can also help children understand that bigger things can happen, which puts a hole in our picture. The death of a loved one like a grandparent or pet creates a hole that takes longer to fill. Allow your child or teenager to talk as much as they want to about the loss. This talking helps the healing process and helps them rebuild their stained-glass picture.

7. Practice gratitude.

In 2020, I was listening to a podcast on *The Daily*, and they were talking about food shortages and food scarcity for families in New York City. There was one food bank where people would get there around three o'clock in the morning and wait in line. They'd wait six, eight, or even twelve hours. When the food came in, they never knew what was going to arrive. It could be a truck full of milk and yogurt, dairy stuff. Or it could be vegetables or bread products that showed up.

They'd stock the shelves, and the customers would come in. They were allowed only so many items. One woman had been there all day waiting and when asked about what she got, with great joy in her voice, she explained how she got chocolate milk and was so excited that it was organic milk for her kids. She also got some organic yogurt for herself and cucumbers, which was one of her favorite foods. She said, "I am so grateful for the opportunity to be here and to get the free food."[11]

How many of us can say we're thankful for our food every day? We might say grace or a blessing before we eat, but are we really thankful for our food? Unlike this woman, most of our kids are complaining about what they have to eat or that it's not enough, or whatever.

I know I'm one of those people. I like my food, but to have that much appreciation for the food she was given and for the people—those who were in line with her and the workers who were bringing up the food—is really just amazing. She was able to reflect upon that and be truly grateful.

8. Take care of yourself.

Remember, a lot of how your kids respond to downers in life depends on how you respond. If you take care of yourself, then that self-care can refresh you, and that gives your child a better chance to do the same thing. So relax and practice self-care.

Also, you just have to be this side of good enough. Life will be what it is in the good times and the bad. When this time of hardship is over, there'll be another one after that. There will also be good times in between, and we just keep unfolding as we go.

9. Teach and practice calming strategies.

Start by brainstorming what helps each family member reduce their stress. Things like deep breathing, listening to music, getting exercise, journaling or drawing emotions, or throwing some cold water on your temples are just a few to get started with. In addition to being a role model for your children, everyone should practice the strategies to be effective in the heat of the moment. If a child hasn't practiced calming breathing techniques, it's not going to work if you tell them to take three deep breaths when they are all worked up.

For more calming strategies, practice techniques, and other ideas to help with long-term stress, check out: Wired and Connected.

CHAPTER 8

FINDING A PURPOSE

"Joy's soul lies in the doing." —William Shakespeare

When we are doing things as humans, we feel great joy and a sense of accomplishment. This is the basis for building a resilient family. First of all, our brains are wired to influence our environment. Humans want and need to be efficacious. It is how we survive. If we were not wired to survive and to be effective, we would not have existed very long as a species.

Children who are in preschool naturally imitate the productive work of their parents. My grandson loves to push our toy mower around the yard. Our granddaughter loves to be the "teacher" while she teaches her younger brother his letters. At school and home (with chores), children are learning how to be efficacious. Children at play are learning how to live socially with others in order to garner success in their activities. In other words, does your child, when faced with a problem, feel like they can face the problem and try to solve it?

When I was first entering middle school, I had a socially disastrous start after losing my two best neighborhood friends since preschool. Rather than going outside to play after school, I spent most of my time eating snacks and watching TV in the basement. Needless to say, I gained a lot of weight.

Thankfully, the school had a sign up in the hall about a new after-school intramural activity: floor hockey. I had never played hockey before, but I thought it sounded pretty fun. So, I recruited my younger brother, and the two of us grabbed some old brooms and a tennis ball and started playing in the basement. I then saved up some money and bought my first hockey stick so that I could join the hockey program. The decision to join changed my life. I went from a husky TV-watching boy to a reasonably fit kid with a bunch of new friends. I played center and goalie throughout middle school and continued playing in a high school league. I even played at the University of Denver.

From a self-efficacy standpoint, I was struck with a problem and found a way to solve it myself. It had nothing to do with my parents stepping in and solving it for me. They did not know anything about playing hockey. I just happened to see the sign and decided to take advantage of the opportunity. I felt my own sense of independence and competence while becoming socially connected at the same time. My self-esteem increased, as well, with all the practicing in our basement and cheering my team on. **Parent overinvolvement does not help children feel efficacious. It is something they need to do for themselves.**

Self-efficacy and the Exceptional Student

Self-efficacy is not only important for all children, but it is essential for exceptional students (i.e., ADHD, learning disabled, temperamental emotions, autism). The best-selling author and advocate for the needs of exceptional students, Dr. Robert Brooks, talks about the concept of helping your child find their island of competence. Even if your child is struggling in school or with their emotions and behavior, it's important for them to focus on their island of competence. Or, as Brooks says, In an "ocean of inadequacy," you need to have "islands of competence."[1]

Over the years, I've had the opportunity to watch many exceptional children find a purpose in their lives that was based on their strengths and unique talents. Take the eighth grader who has severe dyslexia. She worked with a learning specialist several days a week at school and had twice weekly after-school tutoring. Her talent, or her island of competence, was dance. This young lady just lived for dancing.

One day, her mother talked to me about how her daughter was still struggling and had concerns about the approaching high school years. She asked me, "Should we take her out of dance so she can do more tutoring?" My answer was, "No!" As far I know, she danced throughout her high school years, and I would not be surprised if she's still dancing today. She needed her dancing island of competence to counterbalance the academic struggles in her life.

Another mother of an exceptional student said to me, "My goal is for her to walk out of school with confidence. I want her to feel like she can solve a problem or that she can get through something that's hard, but she doesn't have to master it. She doesn't have to be perfect at it. I'd much rather have her confidence intact walking out of school, than feeling like she was a failure because she wasn't at a certain level." This is a great example of a sense of self-efficacy.

Another student, who was a rather tall fifth-grade boy, lacked any sort of self-efficacy or purpose with school. His response to academic challenges was simply to put his head down on the table and refuse to work. One day the teacher put a test paper on his desk. The fifth grader's response was to simply tear it up in front of her. The teacher called the principal who came in and had to wrestle this student out of the room.

I knew that his island of competence and passion was fly fishing. For our final session, years later, I took him to a local lake. Following his guidance, we caught dozens of blue gills on our fly rods while my preschool son brought them in with his net. We must have caught and released thirty of them.

Some fifteen years later, I ran into his mother. After I asked how he was doing, she said, "He's a fly-fishing guide in Montana and loving it." His island of competence became his purpose in life.

Finding a Purpose in Hard Times

Children and teens need a sense of purpose in good times and especially during hard times. In my assessment, the kids who were doing the best during the lockdown and throughout the first year of the pandemic were the ones who took on new hobbies or who ratcheted up their existing hobbies.

One high school student had already been an avid mountain biker. During the lockdown, he learned how to repair bikes and set up a small shop in his parent's garage. Financially, that was a very good decision because at that time you couldn't find a repair shop without a month's wait. Everyone seemed to be getting out on their bikes again. Fortunately for me, I became his first customer when I blew out my rear axle on my road bike. He had it fixed in a week.

When I was on my bike rides, I cannot tell you how many chalk drawings I saw on sidewalks and driveways. Young children were finding a purpose in cheering up others with rainbows and butterflies during some very dark days. My favorites were the ones with inspirational messages, such as, "Keep on going" and "You can make it." That was great inspiration for all of us in surviving the pandemic, as well as for those of us who were pedaling up the hills.

About a month into the lockdown, I was teaching a brain-based Zoom class for my fourth graders. One of the students said, "You have to see what Michael is doing!" Michael turned his lens to a large dry erase board behind him. Excitedly he said, "I'm mapping out the whole brain and want to figure out how it all works!" What a great purpose for him and a great compliment for me as his teacher.

One of my teens at the office used his extra time during the pandemic to complete his Eagle Scout project, which was building a wooden staircase that wound up the hill at a nearby elementary school. A year later, I had the honor of attending his Eagle Court of Honor.

Our teen daughter started with painting her room and then her furniture. Later, she learned how to reupholster furniture. After doing a great job on our kitchen counter stools, she took on reupholstering several of our office sofas.

The Growing Together Project

In the fall of 2021 when we returned to meeting in person, I led an activity for all of the preschool and kindergarten through eighth grade classrooms called Growing Together. I purchased some hand-shaped cutouts in a variety of colors. I then went to each class and asked them five questions (for younger grades, I shortened it to one or two questions) and instructed them to draw a picture or write the answer to one of the questions. The five questions were:

1. What's something you liked about the pandemic? *Most of these answers were about being home with mom and dad.*

2. What's something new that you learned to do during the pandemic? *The responses included an amazing list of purpose-driven behaviors.*

3. How did you help your family or community during the pandemic? *The number one response for younger children was "wearing a mask so people didn't get sick." For the older students, it was "helping my family or my neighbors."*

4. What was hard for you? *Younger students answered, "Wearing masks" and older students answered, "Being away from friends."*

5. What did you learn about yourself as you overcame those difficulties and how could this help you in your future? *The number one theme was "learning that I could handle more than I thought was possible."*

After the students were finished drawing or writing on their hand cutouts, I put them up in each classroom with all the fingers pointing inward, creating a large circle of hands. As we talked about being resilient, I told the students, "We all grew together. When you drop a teacup, what happens? It breaks. When you drop a rubber ball, what happens? It bounces back."

These new purposes gave the students a sense of independence, self-efficacy, and self-confidence. Doing this exercise is so much more worthwhile for child and teen development during hard times than spending hours on end doing online gaming or social media.

Finding a Purpose in Free Play

In their best-selling book, *The Coddling of the American Mind,* authors Greg Lukianoff and Jonathan Haidt talk about the decline in free play since the 1980s (due to fears of child kidnapping) and the rise in competition for admission to top universities. In addition, we can't forget about the trauma and fears that teens face from the endless cycle of school shootings since Columbine High School.

We know from the research that the time children and teens spend in free play activities (especially outdoors) has been plummeting over the last several decades. There is a plethora of additional explanations for this, including increased homework demands, structured sports, electronics, social media, and increasing fears about childhood safety.

Wired and Connected covers the loss of free play in more detail and talks specifically about the work of Lenore Skenazy. In short, Skenazy and her "Let Them Play" organization promote giving children more free playtime and letting them discover new purposes. She tells parents to think about one thing you used to do as a child but are now worried about your child doing.

Besides simply playing without adults directing the activities, Skenazy wants you to think about various purpose-driven activities that kids took on during the pandemic. She recommends sitting down with your child and mapping out a list of purpose-driven activities for them to try, such as walking the dog, cooking a family dinner, or riding a bike to their friend's house, all of which offer opportunities to solve problems and overcome new challenges.[2]

Thinking back to my own childhood, I loved the challenges of collecting refundable soda bottles in the ditches so we could buy nickel candy at the store. In fifth grade, I learned a lot about woodworking with my own power tools and the value of hard work when I grew my own garden in the backyard. My mom gave me permission that year to paint the logo of the St. Louis Blues hockey team on my bedroom wall. I also learned from my father to not do a half-assed job the first time I wanted to wash his car and mow the lawn. While not every woodworking model turned out well and not every plant survived in the garden, I was learning how to handle frustration and overcome obstacles on my own.

Experiences Build Resiliency

At times, your child will experience something that you will find distressing, but you cannot just give up on these opportunities. Our daughter walked our dogs around the local park for years. One day, she came home and told me how some boys were driving by and started commenting on her body. While I had a visceral pain for her, I explained that these were called catcalls and were disgusting. We then talked about staying on the canal path where lots of families walk rather than looping around onto the street sidewalk.

It is much better to let your child discover new realities and struggle with problem-solving when the consequences of making a mistake are much smaller than later in life when the consequences are much greater.

In *The Coddling of the American Mind,* Lukianoff and Haidt also trace the history of overprotective parenting and the lack of unstructured activities for children and younger teens. They found that college students who struggle with solving problems without parental support also struggle with taking on challenging topics and points of view, which make them feel uncomfortable. Obviously, these are not examples of resilient children and teens.

Shame-Free Parenting Tips for Overcoming Resistance

What if you have a child who is resistant to trying new activities or searching for a new purpose? There are many parents who offer all sorts of new opportunities, but their child or teen says no. As we have explored in previous chapters, the addiction to gaming and social media are very hard to break. Here are some thoughts which may help break some repetitive behaviors.

1. Utilize blocks of time.

When building structure around electronics and social media, create a block of time for those activities, separated by blocks of time for IRL activities. Another words, if they want the gaming, they must do some other activities.

2. Come from their needs base.

While you have the need for your child to find new purposes and learn to be more resilient, that might not be what they are looking for. So, you have to really think about what is the carrot that will motivate your child. Even if it is not in your value system, you might decide to let them get a Nerf gun if that's what their buddies are into. If need be, you can even offer extra screen time in exchange for a new activity.

3. Brainstorm activities.

Sit down with your child (or have them do it on their own) and just start mentioning the entire plethora of opportunities that could be available. When recently brainstorming activities with a family of a middle school student who was obsessed with gaming, the kid's face finally lit up when I said camping. His dad was on board, so they practiced camping in the back yard, spent many fun hours shopping for gear, and took two trips that summer.

4. Do it together or have them do it themselves.

It's perfectly fine to do some things together if that is the support your child needs. For our daughter, we found that doing some things together made it much more enjoyable for her because she's an intensely social person and wants to talk while doing things. You don't want your child to be dependent on you all of the time, so also have them try some new activities with a sibling or some friends.

5. Find other groups if the activity is out of your comfort zone.

My father's idea of camping was staying in a three-star hotel, and my mother never went camping when she was growing up. So, on my own, I asked to join Boy Scouts. I can still remember the evening before my first camping trip. I sat on the bedroom floor surrounded by all my equipment and went down the checklist that was in the scout manual. To this day, I love to camp, and I guide my life and business with checklists.

6. Let go of your fears.

Perhaps your child wants to ride their bike to a friend's house that is several miles away. Crossing major intersections is a cause of concern for all parents, but rather than cancelling your child's desire outright, try riding the route together the first time or two. Then go halfway with them and have the friend meet you in the middle. Before long, your child will be happily riding back and forth. Think of this as good training for your teen driving a car someday.

7. Consider your child's exceptional needs.

Some children have more anxious temperaments and will need to take things in small chunks. All it takes is some success with an activity or a big smile and then they will be ready for more. However, children with ASD often struggle with trying new things. The etiology of this is their inability to paint a picture of what this new thing might be like in their minds. Start by reviewing something they have already experienced in life and then extrapolate how this new thing will be fairly similar. You might also want to explore activities offered by groups who are familiar with ASD.

8. Be open to lots of alternative activities and experiences.

I had two students who were more introverted socially and were not into many of the traditional activities that their more extroverted peers were into. Both, however, loved to read and write. So, their new activity was to write a book together. Some other possible activities might involve electronics. I had a sixth grader who was really interested in the stock market. He had his own portfolio and spent time researching companies to invest in. His goal was to save money for college. Another one of my middle school students became interested in exploring real estate opportunities. I encouraged him to find some kind of group chat around real estate so that there would be a social component to his purpose.

CHAPTER 9

ADVENTURES

What do you think of when you hear the word *adventure*? Perhaps you think back to some special times in your childhood or maybe an adventure your family had pre-COVID. Or maybe you were all dreaming about a future adventure during the pandemic to help you get through the tough days. I had promised my daughter a trip to see the Harry Potter tour at the Warner Brothers Studio outside London at the end of eighth grade. Then COVID hit in the spring of her eighth grade year, and we had to wait until August of 2022 to take the trip. Thankfully, it was worth the wait.

I asked my podcast producer, Sydney, what she thought about when she heard the word *adventure*. I loved her answer: "As a mom with three kids of very different ages, I think about spending time with each child individually. To be able to devote a whole weekend to just hang out, go to dinner, go for a hike, or just do what they want to do would be special—just the two of us."

What might some of those adventures be? She continued, "Our preschooler loves tornadoes. When it gets cloudy, my husband and I get him in the car, and we just drive around looking at the clouds. We don't know where we are going, but we just follow the clouds. He also loves those bright advertising spotlights way up in the sky. We will take off and try to find them. We never know where we might end up. It's a magical time for us." Thankfully, we do not have many tornadoes in the middle of Denver.

What Makes For A Good Adventure?

As we can see from Sydney's experience, adventures are not something you do every day (although you can find an adventure in every day of your life) so that makes them feel different and special to your children. Many times, adventures are things you are trying for the first time, which means heightened emotions.

There is also the element of spontaneity (like clouds appearing) along with a good dose of single-mindedness as a family, meaning, you are not trying to multitask, not doing too many different things at the same time. You are just focused on your adventure. That also means turning off your own devices and being focused on your children.

Another tip from Sydney is that the adventure is not totally planned out and they never really know where they might end up. Adventures might have some sort of goal in mind, but you do not have to have every detail planned out. As they used to say in the sixties, "You have to go with the flow." According to Sydney, "It's like chasing a rainbow. You never know where your adventure will take you."

Some COVID Adventures

When the lockdown began in March of 2020, it was amazing how quickly people around the world found ways to turn the experience into an adventure of sorts. Families with young ones started going on teddy bear hunts (i.e., looking for teddy bears that others were putting in their front windows). Italy had some great news clips of people throwing their windows open at sunset and having grand sing-alongs. Here in the United States, families came out to their front porches at eight o'clock every evening to clap, howl, or cheer as a show of solidarity for health care workers and first responders. I fired off some fireworks one night, but my wife quickly put an end to that. Despite all the suffering that came with COVID, it was like the whole world found a way to emotionally support others in creative ways.

About the third week of the lockdown, my daughter agreed to go on a bike ride with me to our local park and have a picnic lunch. We went to the very middle of the park, away from the trees, and spread out our blanket. After eating, we just stretched out on the grass and stared up at the blue sky with hardly anyone around us. At that moment I thought, "How often does a dad get to have a weekday picnic with his teen daughter?" I felt so blessed.

After moving to Zoom therapy sessions, I quickly began hearing stories from children and parents about some of the adventures they had been on. My favorite was from a family who lives in a small mountain town in southwestern Colorado. It was still late winter there, but the dad decided to pull out the summer camper, throw some blankets in, and load up his two sons. He drove into the woods for about half a mile before he had to stop because of the snow. They made dinner on the stove, and then snuggled on the camper bed and watched a family movie on the disc player. Later, as the youngest one fell asleep, he drove them back home to bed.

An Adventure Can Be Anything

While most of the adventures I like to talk about are in the outdoors (*Wired and Connected* has lots of research on how being outside is good for our physical and mental health, including lower blood pressure, lower levels of stress hormones, improved immune system functioning, and better sleep), adventures don't have to take place outside. One father I know was frustrated because his son never took interest in the things he liked to do outside. They had a motor home, dirt bikes, and jet skis. His son just wasn't interested and only wanted to be involved with computers. Their adventure together was getting in line at five o'clock in the morning at a local mall, in order to be the first ones in the Apple Store for the newest iPad.

You also do not have to wait until your kids are older. Just walking to the park with my two-year-old grandson is an adventure in itself. In past outdoor adventures with my preschool son, I used to bring along lunch and our small tent. We would stop, eat, and then have nap time. Nothing is better than just lying there watching the innocence and peacefulness of your child sleeping.

We also had a little ritual when he would wake up. I'd say, "Are you awake?" He would reply, "Yes, are you awake?" I'd answer, "Yes," and then would ask, "Are you ready to do something?" He'd say, "Yes," and would then ask, "Are *you* ready to do something?" Then off we'd go.

By having adventures at different ages with your child, you get to watch them grow in size and ability as well as in their problem-solving skills. As parents, you must remember that despite your anxieties, your children can handle more than you think they can. You just need to bite your tongue and give them the chance to demonstrate what they can do.

For my son, it was not too long before he was coming up with a better way to hang a bear bag (a bag that holds your food at night when you are camping and is strung up in a tree) than how I was doing it and was matching me step-for-step as we hiked a 14,000-foot mountain. I'll never forget the first time he led me up the mountain as a young teen. When he was younger, I'd always lead him on our scuba diving trips. On our most recent trip to Iceland, I followed him as we descended over a shelf into the dark water below. I was now feeling comforted by him leading me.

Shame-Free Parenting Tips for Planning an Adventure

1. Consider age-appropriate adventures.

Children preschool age and younger can be quite difficult when you try to spontaneously plan an adventure. For these ages, start with a couple of things that you know they will reasonably enjoy and then add some structure to it.

You can do this by telling them what you will be doing on a given day (i.e., "Tomorrow we are going to swim at the lake for our adventure time and then we will do a bike ride the following day.") As they get older, you can then add more spontaneity, brainstorming, and mutual planning.

2. Have a flexible mindset.

When it comes to selecting adventures, as the parent, you will need to suspend some of your own desires. You have to be flexible in what you do based on the varying desires of your children. You might be able to find a creative way to blend your desires together.

For instance, my daughter was a first grader when she first joined our family. At that time, I was so excited to take her on our annual pumpkin picking trip at a friend's farm (we usually collect about fifty pumpkins for our church's volunteer program). She quickly explained that she didn't want to do that. Fortunately, I remembered that there was a Claire's store right off the highway on our pumpkin route. After picking the pumpkins (and she was nothing but smiles), we went on our first adventure to Claire's. Covered in dirt and mud, we both had fun browsing through all the merchandise. Years later, we repeated a Claire's adventure when she got her ears pierced. Not fond of needles, she asked me to hold her hand through the procedure. That's pretty special for a dad.

A flexible mindset also means that you put some of your needs for the adventure on hold while you focus on your child. I have had season tickets to the University of Colorado football games for almost forty years, and I love to watch every play of every game. When we took our preschool-aged son to his first game, we spent hours doing pre-game activities like seeing Ralphie the Buffalo, following the marching band to the stadium, getting snacks, collecting pom poms during the cheerleader sing-along, and then watching Ralphie run onto the field. It was amazing. When I was finally able to sit down to watch the game, I quickly realized that I didn't get to watch many of the plays and that required me to be flexible with my game watching mindset.

3. Be creative and resilient as problems arise.

Having a flexible mindset means weathering problems that emerge on an adventure. Part of being a resilient family means that you find ways to have fun with creative adventures, even in the toughest of times. Now that the pandemic has passed us by, it is important for families to bond while learning to handle the problems that can arise on any great adventure.

What is the key to encountering problems on an adventure?

First, stay calm. In scuba diving, when you face a problem, the first thing to do is relax. Rather than getting upset and uptight about the problem, teach your child to stay calm and realize that things will be okay.

Next, engage your child in problem-solving. Just like our children often help us with technology issues, engage them when you need to solve a problem. I cannot tell you how many times I have relied on my son or daughter to come up with a solution that I never would have thought of. (To this day, I am so thankful for my son's problem-solving skills when determining which path we should take while we were backpacking in the Utah desert.)

In addition, never be afraid to ask complete strangers for help. Adventures mean that you are being open to what's presented to you and open to the world around you. As my father used to say, "Everyone wants to help. You just have to ask them." Despite all the negative things in the news, this is the opportunity to teach your child that the majority of the people in the world are just like them. **Empathy and help surround us.**

4. Embrace ambiguity.

During COVID, we all had to embrace the ambiguity of not knowing what was coming next. We had to accept new realities day by day and adjust our behavior accordingly. It is the same thing with adventures; and it is this change of plans that makes your family more resilient.

In having a flexible adventure mindset, you will quickly discover that Plan B is often better than Plan A would have ever been. After our train was late to Brussels and we missed the connection to Amsterdam, my daughter discovered that sitting on the floor between two train cars with a group of strangers was way more fun than sitting inside the luxury of the train car. It is all about embracing the process of adventures.

5. Get out of the resorts.

In her book *Unselfie,* Michelle Borba discusses how important it is to get kids out of their normal circumstances and experience how others live.

For many American families, going to the all-inclusive resorts on the beaches of Mexico is great family bonding time. For kids, you can have your hair braided and all the virgin daiquiris and snacks you want. If you just fly in and out of the airport and go directly to the resort, what do your kids think about Mexico? To them, it's all rainbows and butterflies because that's all they have experienced.

Borba's book discusses the research on having wealth and empathy. While you might think that having great resources translates to greater empathy, it is the exact opposite. The more people have, the more they want to maintain their lifestyle and actually give less to the well-being of others compared with families who do not have as much.

To change perceptions of the world, you have to expose your kids to how others live so they can feel empathy and then work to help a world in need. While my family and I have had great trips to Mexico and many other places, I have always tried to spend some time out of the resort and expose my kids to the true reality of others. This might be as simple as traveling through the local countryside on the way to your destination and talking about the living conditions of those who live outside of the resorts.

Excursions like eco-trips can also help your children think about nature and the destruction of the environment. Many teens have had life-changing experiences on class trips to poverty-stricken areas in order to build houses or install water systems. If you do not get out of the resorts, however, your kids will never experience the realities of how most people live.

When you get home, spend some time as a family talking about all the great fun but also how your child might want to get involved in helping others. My son and I have a new understanding of abject poverty after we rode in a cab through Addis Ababa, Ethiopia.

6. Find low-cost options.

Remember that you do not have to go far or spend lots of money to have great adventures. Taking your kids to a drive-in movie theatre or going crawdad fishing in a nearby creek are also great adventures. In addition, just planning and preparing for an adventure can be a lot of fun.

Many times, fun adventures also just happen in the middle of normal life. Any time the power went out during the winter, my dad would start up the fireplace and mom would gather all seven of us for warmth and time together. While we kids were always excited when the power came back on, my mom was always disappointed. If she had it her way, she would have left the power off all night long.

7. Be spontaneous.

An amazing core of Zen philosophy is the line, "Not knowing is most intimate." When every detail is perfectly planned out, you are basically trying to control your anxiety from what *might happen* on an adventure or trip. While reducing anxiety, detailed planning cuts you off from being intimate with your own vulnerability and the vulnerability that your family feels as you bond together in the uncertainty of your adventure.

Traveling with children does mean you need the supplies, equipment, and food for any adventure you go on (that's why I love the new luggage wagons that parents are pulling through the parks). It is not the same as an Australian college-aged student with a rucksack on a walkabout.

Once you have the equipment, loosely plan your adventure and leave plenty of room for spontaneity. That looseness means taking advantage of opportunities as they arise. (Did you know that turkeys sleep together in treetops? We discovered that when we took up an offer to visit a rancher's property after talking to him at a breakfast diner.)

When you do not have everything planned out perfectly, the beauty of a spontaneous mindset means that you will encounter difficulties along the way. While these can be frustrating, they also provide some fun problem-solving opportunities for your family.

One hot summer day in southern Kentucky, my son and I decided to see how far a Prius could go on the electric battery after it ran out of gas. It wasn't very far. Stranded on the side of the road with no cell service, we got out his little green army men and played in the dirt of a farmer's field. After about an hour, a state trooper pulled up and gave us a gallon of gas. While things didn't go exactly as planned, it was an amazing experience together.

As with other adventures already mentioned, these are things you do not usually do in your day-to-day life. So much of our lives are run by routines (it's the brain's way of saving energy when we do repetitive tasks). After you've become an experienced skier, for example, you do not have to think about it so much. You just get in a flow.

While having routines is beneficial, they become simple repetitions without the awareness we bring to something new or special. So many of my memories from childhood are not from the birthday parties or other annual events, but just simple times where we were in a zone and aware of something beyond our daily routines.

8. Remember the Gottman principles.

Dr. John Gottman, an American psychologist and leader in couples-based therapy, developed seven principles for building healthy relationships. One of them has to do with positive experiences to balance out negative ones. His ideal ratio is 5 to 1.[1] That is, if you have five positive experiences together it will balance out one negative experience. Your family adventures offer a plethora of positive experiences. When you hit the teen years, you will truly understand how adventures can heal your parent-teen relationship.

9. Create rituals.

I want to briefly mention the importance of family rituals. *Wired and Connected* has a whole section on having daily, weekly, monthly, or yearly activities. Think of bedtime rituals, weekend rituals such as a family game night, monthly volunteer opportunities, or yearly adventure activities. (We love to cut down a Christmas tree every year.)

The benefits of rituals are at the core of resiliency. When looking at adults who were raised in alcoholic families, those families that observed rituals and traditions throughout the year were much more resilient as adults compared with families that did not create family rituals. In a sea of chaos, those rituals were things they could count on.

Rituals can be done with extended family or with your friends. Through middle school, my son and I went on an annual float trip with two other dads and their sons. Every summer we would go on increasingly more intense rafting trips. For my daughter, we started going on an annual parent-daughter camping trip when she was in the third grade. Sadly, COVID ended these trips when she finished eighth grade.

10. Have a sense of awe.

Adventures can help you and your child experience a sense of awe. Experiencing awe is good for your mental health. Humans experience awe when something so amazing and so vast happens that challenges our sense of place in the world or makes us question how something is actually done. Seeing a Van Gogh painting, visiting the Anne Frank house, touring a Grand Cathedral, and even looking at the actual Hogwarts castle can produce these emotions.

Going into nature can very much inspire your sense of awe. Maybe it is seeing the Grand Canyon or getting out of the city lights and looking up at the vastness of the universe. My two favorite night sky memories include winter camping at 12,000 feet and floating in the ocean after completing a night dive with my son in the Florida Keys.

For a whole list of adventure activities and more tips on creating adventures, check out my website: adventuredad.org.

CHAPTER 10

VOLUNTEERISM

This book is filled with lots of strategies and tips for parenting through the developmental stages of childhood, but all these strategies serve a larger purpose: **to help children and families be of service to the world community.** It is the same purpose that the term *self-esteem* was designed to accomplish.

Our brains are wired to imitate each other and feel what the other person feels. When someone smiles and says, "Thank you so much," the person being spoken to smiles automatically in response. This, in turn, activates our positive emotions as if we were the receiver. The loop of positivity is absolutely wired in.

The positivity loop has a two-fold benefit in terms of family resiliency. First, you and your child will feel more positive, and feeling positive will boost your resiliency during hard times. Second, the receiver feels a jolt of surprise and happiness, which helps them feel more resilient.

If you followed the pre-pandemic "pay it forward" movement, you know that giving and acts of kindness can spread like wildfire, which makes the entire community—and the entire world—more resilient.

Finding Ways to Give, Even In Isolation

I'd like to start with my own mother, as she is my role model for caring, kindness, and living life to the fullest. At the age of ninety-four, during COVID, she was locked in her retirement community for months at a time through the first year of the pandemic. She entertained herself with books and watching sports on TV (she's a big Kansas City Chiefs football fan), but since she was not able to participate in the retirement community's voluntary activities as they had been cancelled, she decided to take up knitting for the first time in her life. My sister taught her the basics and dropped off the supplies for her. My mother began knitting six by six inch squares out of the yarn. She's made batches of these squares. My sister then mailed them off to a nonprofit organization, which made the squares into blankets for the homeless.

Knitting the squares occupied her mind during the long period of isolation and brought her great joy that she could still help others. While she will never see or meet the recipients of those blankets, her mirror neuron system was activated just by visualizing the recipient receiving her gift.

As the news coverage of COVID grew during the first several weeks, it was not long before news stations and social media were covering the many acts of charity people were doing to help their communities (thereby helping themselves). We all started thinking about the needs and vulnerability of the elderly. Given how full of people the grocery stores were, many families took on the task of shopping for their elderly neighbors.

Our daughter continued the shoe drive that her school had started right before the break. Every day she checked the trash can for any donations of gently used shoes. Sure enough, she filled up several trash cans full of shoes. She felt great joy as she bundled them up in trash bags and we dropped them off outside the school's front door.

I was very impressed hearing about a volunteer in New York City—a man who helped out at a food pantry. Every day he would drive to grocery stores to collect close to expiring foods and collected some eight tons of food. He would pull up to the food bank, have the truck unloaded, and be gone in forty-five minutes. That food bank served fifteen thousand people every week.

Colorado Rooted

I would like to share a story of one high school student because his volunteer service has so many valuable lessons. At the time I interviewed him over the phone, Harrison Cymbala was in his senior year and getting ready to go to college. He described to me how he created a program called Colorado Rooted: "Our main goal is to improve the environment I grew up in and that I'm so passionate about." He and a few friends started selling merchandise and accepting online donations in order to buy and plant tree saplings at nearby parks and green spaces. When COVID hit, they were not able to get together or promote their program in-person anymore and had to make a change.

Harrison told me, "We couldn't keep doing things the way we had, so we pivoted in the moment and developed a new product. We knew that people wanted to get outside more, and we wanted to promote people getting out into their yards and gardening. Not everyone knew what to do or wanted to go out shopping. So, we designed the Garden in a Box as a solution. Everything you need comes in a box so that people can get outside and not have to try and shop for everything." Harrison and his group of friends developed several types of gardens available for purchase.

He explained further, "We have your basic Garden in a Box with a variety of vegetables. We also have a salsa box with different types of peppers, tomatoes, and spices so that people can make their own salsa. We also have an urban garden box that comes with a pre-made bowl that already has lettuce growing in it. It also comes with a variety of herbs for making your own salad. If an online order for a garden box comes in locally, we will deliver it to the person's doorstep. If it's from further away, we mail it out the very next day."

The business grew and grew, especially after Colorado Rooted was featured on a podcast in Boulder, Colorado. At the end of our interview, I asked him two questions. First, I asked if he had a green thumb. His answer: "I'm not big into gardening myself. That's not my specialty, but it is my mom's. I have always grown up having gardens at our house and my mom really enjoys it."

My second question was about what he was planning on for college. As you might guess, he said, "The program I'm going into has a big emphasis on nonprofit organizations. I'll make a lot of connections there that will be good for my personal growth and for the growth of our organization. I'm looking forward to taking it even further."

As we signed off, I had one more comment for Harrison, "As social gatherings are coming back, I'm picturing a bunch of teenagers in a garage, putting these boxes together, and having a lot of fun."

His answer: "Yes, it's always a lot of fun."

What could be better? Volunteering is also a way to have fun.

Takeaways

As I took another look at my interview with Harrison, I came up with some key takeaways for you, your family, and your children.

1. Colorado Rooted emerged from Harrison's environmental experiences and his mother's role modeling of being outside in her garden. These came together in a deep passion to help the environment and help others get outside.

2. Think about the amount of time Harrison and his friends had to spend planning and creating their first product.

3. When COVID hit, they had to pivot. Every business in the world was talking about how they could possibly pivot during times of hardship. His group looked at customer desires and COVID realities and found their niche.

4. Think about the valuable problem-solving lessons Harrison and his friends learned on the way. Not to mention having to hold meetings on Zoom.

5. Think about the financial experience Harrison and his friends gained. Learning how to raise funds is invaluable experience. Then, throw in a good dose of expense estimates, price setting, and shipping management.

6. There is also the component of learning how to assert one-self with adult customers while learning about customer satisfaction.

7. Think about the many positive social experiences Harrison and his friends were having during the pandemic. So many other teens were in their rooms on social media and gaming, or hooking up in a park to smoke marijuana.

8. Harrison took his passion and his purpose on to college where he may very well have a career in serving others through a nonprofit organization.

What parent would not want their teen to have these experiences?

Off air, I asked Harrison if he had ever heard of Victory Gardens. He had not. I had great joy explaining how, almost exactly one hundred years ago, the world was experiencing the Spanish Flu pandemic. It was also WW I, and US citizens were asked to grow their own gardens so as to have more food to send to our troops. It seems like resiliency repeats itself throughout history.

Volunteering Feeds Your Soul

For the past thirty-nine years, my family has voluntarily been running a program for mental health consumers (adults with debilitating mental health problems). I've watched both of my younger children grow up at the program. Each year, they took on more and more volunteer responsibilities. You truly have never heard a more enthusiastic bingo caller than our youngest daughter.

One of my favorite monthly gatherings is when we do talent nights (i.e., our guests get up and perform). The participants are so eager and excited to get up and sing, recite poetry, tell jokes, or play instrumentals. They are completely excited to share their talents because no one else in their life ever asks them what they have to offer others.

All too often, we are too busy in our lives with work, school, sports, arts, family activities, and just putting food on the table. We often feel stressed when we are asked to take on additional responsibilities. These are legitimate issues in today's fast-paced world. Take a moment to think about what's worse: deciding to give a little bit more or living a life where nobody thought you had anything of importance to offer.

We all know that self-care is important, and the beauty of volunteering to help those in need is that it will feed your soul and nourish your mental health. I personally find great solace and motivation in one of my favorite sayings: "Life is short, and pain is long. We were put here for one thing, to help each other." I've been through some personally and professionally rough times—times you couldn't pay me enough to relive. These words keep me going as much as our program for mental health consumers does. Volunteering to help others recharges me mentally and emotionally every month.

Shame-Free Parenting Tips to Get Your Family Involved in Volunteer Activities

1. Think about the empathy system of your unique child.

Some children naturally observe and read nonverbal cues and then have the appropriate emotional response to those observations. Others might struggle with knowing how to observe or taking the time to observe what others are thinking and feeling. Children with ASD or impulsive, hyperactive children will need you to say, "Stop and think about what is going on."

Also keep in mind that there is a difference in the empathy systems between boys and girls, especially after puberty. Extra time will be needed to coach males along this path, and they might do better with more specific hands-on tasks, which you can emotionally process with them afterwards.

Designated roles are also helpful with ASD students or children who struggle with social anxiety.

2. Keep age in mind.

Elementary students can be so sweet and sincere in their desires to help others. Early puberty, however, means a drop in empathy levels with all those hormones and desires to fit in with peers. Don't be too shocked when your middle school student makes a horrible joke about a person in need.

High school students, like our friend Harrison, can be tremendously motivated to make changes in the world. They may, however, not be so wild about participating with their parents. The solution is to invite their friends along or have them take ownership of their own volunteer activities.

3. Start with your child's interests or observations.

When selecting a volunteer opportunity, start with your child's interests, from things they have observed or experienced in real life. As mentioned earlier, travel can be a great way for your children to realize others' needs in the world and form a desire to make a difference in some way. The added benefit is that when we see others in need, whiny and demanding children can begin to gain a better perspective of how they are blessed.

You can also start with some of your own family's struggles. Many a health care or human services worker entered into their careers because of trauma or losses at home. Today, climate change is motivating many young volunteers and entrepreneurs.

4. Explore what your child is learning at school.

One innovative father realized how much carbon was being released every day while parents waited in the carpool line with their engines running. He reached out to the teacher who was teaching about pollution and the children all put up handwritten signs with pictures about turning off your engine. By the end of the year, they had cut the number of idling cars in half.

5. Look to larger needs.

Help your children extrapolate beyond their family's or friend's needs. I do an activity with kindergarten students where I begin passing out small oranges. Some get one, some might get two or three, and some do not get any after I run out. Every time I have done this experiment, the children who have more immediately start passing their extra oranges to their friends who don't have any. I always praise them for their great empathy.

We then talk about how those in need might be children in downtown Denver or in other countries around the world. While we do not know them and cannot see them, we should still express our empathy. We also talk about how this relates to food waste in our cafeteria or how our canned food drive will help people whom we will never see. The beauty, I explain, is that we will still feel great about helping.

6. Connect with other charities.

You might also wish to connect with charitable activities that are being directed by your child's school or your faith community. That gives you and your children the joy of sharing empathy with friends.

Over the past twenty-five years, I have watched our school raise hundreds of thousands of dollars for crisis needs around the world. All that money comes in the form of pennies, nickels, dimes, and quarters that the children bring from home. Even better, the kids love the competition as we see which class can bring in the most money.

7. Support your child's motivations.

Occasionally, especially with older children, you might find that their desires to get involved might be challenging your own values and behavior. You might be a sportsman whose child or teen wants to get involved in sensible gun legislation. Or you might be a pro-choice social activist whose teen wants to get involved in the pro-life movement.

While these are hard issues that can drive a huge wedge in a family, my advice is to support your child's motivation. As a parent, you have to ask yourself, "Do I want to raise a child who will think exactly like I do? Or is it more important for them to learn how to think for themselves and be willing to act even when it doesn't agree with me?" Engage your child in calm, logical discussions about all issues.

8. Attend regularly.

Pick a volunteer activity that you can reliably attend. You know your family life. There is no point signing up for a weekly activity when you know how your household roles will prohibit the active involvement you wish. Changes in sports schedules, for instance, can destroy your best intentions.

9. Give financially.

Talk to your kids about financial giving. It has been said that you can contribute your time, your sweat, or your money. Ask yourself which of these categories your family can plug into.

As for financial giving, set aside some money that you, as a family, can decide on where to contribute. Take some time to do some research on the charities your children are interested in. Help them visualize how that money will be spent. For older ones, research what percentage of your donation will go to programming.

10. Focus on integrity.

In an article about teaching integrity to children, author Julie Stevens wrote, "Find ways to nurture your own and your kid's best self. The root of the word *integrity* suggests the psychological process of integrating our inner and outer lives—consciously creating consistency between our conduct and the values to which we aspire. To support this integration for you and your kids, reflect on how your emotions manifest in your behavior and be open to other points of view."[1]

Manifesting your empathetic emotions in volunteer service helps you and your children live out the best version of yourselves.

CHAPTER 11

WHAT DO YOU WANT TO KEEP FROM HARDSHIP? (THERE WILL BE OTHER ZOMBIES.)

When I think of my Growing Together Project, I remember the list of things the children said they liked during the pandemic. First, so many of them loved spending more time with you, their parents. I cannot tell you how many parents I talked to who appreciated slowing down during the lockdown. They were free from the endless task of shuttling their kids back and forth between all their activities. While current research shows some academic delays during the pandemic, wasn't it nice to have a break from the nightly homework routine?[1] Do we really want to go back to overwhelmed schedules and living life at a breakneck pace?

While academic development took a hit, there were plenty of positive outcomes that emerged from the past several years. For marital relationships, the initial research shows that rather than suffering, relationships got better. Pre-COVID, 40 percent of American couples felt their marriage was in trouble. After COVID, it dropped to 29 percent. And 51 percent of respondents reported that they felt more appreciative of their partner and felt a deeper commitment to them.[2] Perhaps togetherness makes the heart grow fonder.

Singles, who were into casual hookups on apps like Tinder, showed a change of heart as well. Research found that people who weren't in a relationship were using dating apps to make "significant connections."[3] Or in other words, someone to bond and connect with.

In Colorado, researchers found positive trends in drug and alcohol use among teens in early July of 2021. Between June 3 and July 3, alcohol use dropped from 29 percent to 21 percent. Electronic cigarette use dropped from 29 percent to 16 percent. Marijuana use dropped from 19 percent to 13 percent, and cigarette use dropped from 8 percent to just 5 percent.[4] While these numbers might have to do with being locked up with the parents versus going out to parties, let's hope that the trends continue.

How Did We Get to Our Pre-COVID Family Life?

In thinking about how to create a resilient family in the future, it might be helpful to look at how we got to where we were pre-COVID. I grew up in the 1960s when our parents valued their own adult relationships with friends. That meant less time focused on just the kids. We were given plenty of freedom but also had fairly strict standards about acceptable behavior and respect for others. We also had plenty of structured routines and rituals that kept us grounded through the hardest of times. Was it all perfect? Certainly not. No style of parenting ever will be.

In the seventies, more and more families had both parents working outside the home. If you look at old *Time* magazines (which I've collected for decades), there were lots of concerns about latchkey kids. These were children who walked home from school and let themselves in the house until their parents came home. While there were obvious concerns about child safety, this generation of kids did learn how to be independent.

In the eighties, there was a big push to focus on child self-esteem. Parents started to focus on being more of a friend to their children instead of just a disciplinarian. While there were some positives in this, parents were concerned about doing anything that might hurt their child's self-esteem.

In the nineties, we saw numerous concerns about entitled teenagers. Lacking stricter rules, socio-economically advantaged teens were spending lots of time and money on themselves and drugs. This was also the time that college acceptance became a bigger concern.

In the two thousands, we saw the trend of helicopter parenting. Homework and academic competition cranked up and parents were obsessed with making sure their child was doing the things they needed to do in order to succeed. When parents weren't involved in academic or athletic demands, there became an obsession with childhood happiness.

In 2010 and the decade that followed, the problem of overparenting became more intense and was epitomized by the term "snow-plow parents." These were parents who were waiting to clear the path of any difficulty their child might face. Family size had been decreasing over the decades before, so parents had more resources and time to focus on just one or two children.

The arrival of social media twisted the realities that kids were exposed to and increased the demand of constant entertainment. Things like family chores and family game nights gave way to homework and retreating into the bedroom with a handheld mobile device. Parents started spending more time on their devices, as well. Parents also started getting more involved in their children's social realities. Pretty soon, rather than recognizing the normal social conflicts that come along with childhood, everything became labeled as bullying.

"Tiger mom" parenting became the new standard with the false belief that parents could "engineer" their child and their child's future. Added to this was the willingness of parents to call out and shame the parenting of others. (As if the stress of parenting wasn't bad enough already!)

Right before COVID, author Michele Borba started talking about "Black Hawk" parents.[5] Cell phone problem-solving became the norm as parents rushed in to take care of their child. If a teen got a B, rather than holding the student accountable, parents were more than happy to call the teacher out. The news outlets covered the phenomenon of parents buying their child into elite colleges.

In her book *Thrivers*, Borba talks about her conversations with five hundred university admission directors. The consensus was that today's college students are extremely academic and have great resumes but are internally empty. Dr. Borba's book discusses internal qualities of success and has great strategies for promoting your child's resilience. If you get a chance, check out my podcast interview with her.[6]

What Did We Learn?

When we experience stress or hardships, such as a global pandemic or a loved one being diagnosed with cancer or dementia, we often start out with a phase of shock and anxiety. In February and March of 2020, we all had an idea that this virus was coming. Clinicians and teachers, trying to reduce student anxieties, were talking to students about this new virus. While reducing the child's anxieties about their danger of getting sick, this also led to anxiety about their older family members.

While still in the initial phase of shock, we began to shelter in place. Our assumptions that this would only last a couple of weeks before we could get back to school, work, and normal life gave way to a longer sense of despair and loss.

As spring wore on, more and more events were cancelled: prom, class trips, graduations, weddings, and sporting events to name a few. As death tolls rose, these losses gave way to anger in our students and families, fueled by the politicizing of the virus. The divided views on how it should be handled left both sides of the fence angry at each other.

Like the summer heat, a sense of inertia started to set in. Adults and students were becoming zombies, feeling forever stuck. "What's the point?" was one of the phrases I heard most frequently from teens.

Some hope began to emerge as the 2020 school year started. While many schools implemented online learning, other schools were at least offering in-school classes either part or full time. For those who were in-person, the new protocols were surreal, but the majority of students were adjusting. My favorite adjustment was a first grader who was swinging a large branch at the other boys. When I asked him why, he replied, "Since we can't touch each other, we use sticks. I thought the branch would really help my team."

"Now that is resiliency!" I thought to myself. The fall of 2020 also brought a hope that this might be over by the holidays.

As January of 2021 rolled more deeply into winter, we all felt the hope slipping away. While lower case numbers in Colorado allowed for some lightening of school protocols, the end of the spring term of 2021 saw a massive wave of students in a mental health crisis. Children's Hospital of Colorado declared a state of emergency.[7] Every therapist in town was booked out for months, and parents struggled to find support.

While things had been looking better, it is when a long-term crisis starts to abate that we more fully begin to assess the damage and losses. It is like when you are struggling in the water, afraid you will drown, and you're just trying to keep your head above water. Later, after finding land again, you sit down, shiver, and think about what could have happened to you.

As summer rolled on, weddings were up again, but so were funerals and memorial services that couldn't take place earlier on. Our hope was building again for in-person school and even the talk of no masks for the kids. All too quickly, however, the Delta variant began to sweep the country. It was another crushing blow.

In the fall of 2021, we were all still holding on with some hope and optimism. As my own school went back, I said to the students, "Well, I got half my wish. We have to wear masks inside, but we do not have to wear them outside! We also have normal class sizes again."

I began talking to all of our students about how we were able to grow together through this hardship with each other's help. We worked on a school-wide project regarding what strengths the students gained from the pandemic that will make them stronger for the rest of their lives (the Growing Together Project discussed in chapter 8).

Now that the pandemic has been officially declared over, on May 11, 2023, we need to remember the concept of **post-traumatic growth**. This means that you can help your child focus on what they learned and how they survived while you also foster their natural sense of hope for the future.

There Will Be Other Zombies

While COVID was a uniquely difficult challenge for our generation of families, we weren't the first ones who have experienced such a calamity. The black death, or bubonic plague pandemic, killed one in four of the people in Europe in the 1300s. Even then, humans kept moving forward despite such amazing loss.

My grandparents survived the Spanish Flu and kept moving forward. When you think about it, the last hundred years alone have witnessed a host of zombie apocalypses. In the United States, we survived two world wars, Vietnam, the Cold War, both Gulf wars and a long war in Iraq and Afghanistan—not to mention 9/11. We've made it through the Great Depression and numerous economic downturns. We've found treatments and cures for many diseases that ravaged our ancestors and have recovered from numerous weather crises. We've even witnessed an attack on our own national Capitol. Still, we've marched on.

While we continue to deal with the scourge of mass shootings, school-based shootings, and are only beginning to tackle climate change, humankind will continue to expand on the progress of past generations. The evolution of a society requires that we continue to seek out those who are oppressed and march toward Civil Rights for all.

In my own lifetime, I've witnessed several civil changes such as the passage of the Civil Rights Act, the Americans with Disabilities Act, Title Nine, and recently the Gay and Interracial Marriage Act. We are now looking at racism in new ways and increasing our awareness of people who identify as LGBTQ+. We are also beginning to address the mental health needs of our children and teens.

Does that mean we have accomplished everything yet? No. In fact, humans will never conquer all of our zombies. It's not possible. Besides COVID, think about the normal changes in life that impact us all. The death of a beloved pet, the passing of a grandparent, a family member with cancer, a death by suicide, and a divorce are just some of the issues I've been helping families with for the past forty years.

While we cannot, nor should we, make life all rainbows and butterflies for our children, it is possible for us to accept suffering, continue on, and foster a new generation of resilient doctors, scientists, engineers, teachers, poets, and philosophers. Right now, our children are learning the hard lessons of life and using their empathy systems to guide their paths into the future.

Life is indeed an amazing hike up a series of very tall mountains. There are moments of great joy when you are walking through a field of flowers, not to mention the awe of looking out from a summit. At the same time, there are many false summits where you realize that you aren't to the top of that mountain yet. In spite of that, after expressing our fatigue and frustration, we gird ourselves and start hiking again.

There will be many zombies along the way that we will need to handle and solve. Hopefully, having survived the COVID-19 pandemic, your children will take their learned problem-solving skills with them. They have been resilient.

As a parent, you cannot be afraid of the zombies. You have to remember that your family story, and your child's story, is like a stained-glass window with tens of thousands of small glass pieces. Good or bad, we are constantly adding in new pieces of glass.

Even when life's challenges shatter our window a bit, we learn to piece it together again. This is who we are. We can't always avoid the shattering of our window as loss is the nature of human life. As stated by Jennifer Frey in her review of the book *Life is Hard: How Philosophy Can Help Us Find Our Way*, "We are born to suffer. But we can still live well, not in spite of our suffering but in full acknowledgment of it."[8]

Follow the Children's Examples

In the fall of 2022, there was a great story about a family who survived the floodwaters in eastern Kentucky. They lost everything. Thanks to the several camping trailers that poured in from around the country, the family was able to stay in a campground. The area was filled with donated lawn chairs, picnic tables, bikes, and toys. Standing next to his two young children, the father said, "My kids are pretty tough, and we've been through a lot."

This story highlights how we, as a society, and communities of people can come together, enact our empathy, and support our survival. Even better is the campground full of toys and bikes because one of the secrets to childhood resiliency is the ability to block out your concerns and just play. For children, playing cures a lot of the world's wounds.

As a father, grandfather, and professional who has worked with children and teens for four decades, despite all the negative news and the massive problems in front of us, I'm still as optimistic as ever. Why? Because I see natural empathy in children every day. I see them laugh every day, and I see them grow and mature into hardworking, conscientious adults. I get to see the hope for our future in each one of them.

As for you, parents of the next generation, **just relax.** Remember, you only have to be this side of good enough. Nature will take care of the rest.

Shame-Free Parenting Tips on Where to Go From Here

Thankfully, modern parenting has more and more brain research on how your child's brain develops. In *Wired and Connected,* I wove the most current brain research into suggestions for parents. Rather than just focusing on childhood happiness, I believe we really need to look at internal development and legitimate parenting strategies.

1. Create an emotional base for empathy.

Start curbing the talk about how special your kids are. While this emotional base is needed through about the age of five, starting kindergarten means realizing that **all children are special.**

Push your child's natural empathy to others, rather than just focusing on themselves. This self-focus will reemerge in the teen years, as they struggle to find their unique talents and abilities. If they have a good base for empathy for others, you'll really help them get through adolescence.

2. Embrace growth opportunities.

Take off the overprotective bubble wrapping. Your child needs more freedom to learn and grow. They also have to face struggles in academics and their social lives. Kids make mistakes, and they need to make mistakes.

Why do we need stress and hardship to grow? When trying to grow trees in the Biosphere 2 project, the trees would grow straight. But when they got taller, they simply fell over due to an underdeveloped root system. What was missing for the tree's survival was wind. It is the hardship of wind that promotes root development.[9] **Resiliency requires hardship.**

Perhaps my favorite sports star quote comes from basketball great Michael Jordan, who said, "I've missed more than 9,000 shots in my career. I've lost almost 300 games. Twenty-six times, I've been trusted to take the game-winning shot and missed. I've failed over and over and over again in my life. And that is why I succeed."[10]

So, next time your child comes to you with a problem (either in-person or on the phone), I want you to take a moment to think about the situation and your child's developmental phase. Ask yourself, "Is this a potential growth opportunity for my child? Will I interfere with their problem-solving by giving them a quick solution?"

If you realize that the answer to these questions is yes, then say, "I have confidence in your ability to solve this problem." Then walk away or end the call before you get sucked back in.

3. Reevaluate your family priorities.

Now that we are on the back end of COVID, take the time to reevaluate your family priorities. Perhaps it's time to take a play out of my mother's parenting handbook. We were allowed to have one night a week for an extracurricular activity. While this hardly seems possible in today's world, perhaps you can trim out just one thing a week and slow down. The faster we spin as a family means less time to stop and think about how you want to be resilient, and pass that resiliency along to your child.

Some of the best memories of my childhood came from the many long car drives we took as a family. There were no electronic screens to entertain us from the more-than-two-thousand-mile trips we went on. We just entertained ourselves by talking and playing car games as a family.

If you are going to allow electronics, I'd highly recommend books on tape or podcasts, such as Jamie Lee Curtis's *Camp Cartwright*. While I never thought I'd enjoy a book involving mermaids, I couldn't have enjoyed it more than when I listened to it with my then sixth-grade daughter on a very long drive to Texas.

4. Learn from life.

In closing, I want to end with the words from children themselves. I love the concept of post-traumatic growth. When I asked several kids what they learned about themselves that can help them in the future, here are some of the things they said:

- I learned to be more grateful.
- I learned to write feelings in story form.
- I learned that watching too much TV makes you feel sick.
- I learned to use plants as a calming technique when stressed.
- I worked hard to achieve personal goals.
- I realized my introversion and optimism.
- I learned that I didn't always need to be so stressed out.
- I took on the challenge of being insecure about myself.
- I learned to embrace being alone and facing the fear of losing family.

These are the life lessons we want to promote each and every day.

ACKNOWLEDGMENTS

My mom is the strongest woman I've ever known. Having been through numerous tragedies in her own life, she continues to greet each day with joy, generosity, and kindness toward others. Her faith in God and the inherent belief in the potential of other human beings are her deepest roots. Roots that she passed on to her five children. I have been blessed by having her same trust that everything will work out. While longing to be with God and my father, she continues to be an inspiration to others. She is the reason I have hope for the future of our children.

At ninety-seven, she, like millions of others, contracted COVID. Fitting with her character, she said to my sister, "Tell everyone not to worry about me." The day after she was admitted to an isolated COVID room, however, she said on the phone to me that she felt so alone in the room (she has always been a very social creature). That cut me to the bone as I thought about my mother dying alone. It's the same feeling tens of millions of families around the world felt when they couldn't be with their loved ones when they left this world.

Thankfully, my mother survived it and is now back at home. I'm grateful to all the doctors, nurses, and first responders who were there for our family members during a global pandemic. They risked their lives to save lives and to bring peace and dignity to those who did not survive.

I appreciate all the families in the world who found resiliency during and after the pandemic. I end each episode of my podcast *(Legit Parenting)* with a segment called "Things of Beauty Make Me Cry." Some of these stories are based on the sheer beauty of human abilities which are truly awe inspiring. Many, however, are based on the resiliency of people during and after times of hardship. Those parents who have had hardships in their families, and yet continue with their commitment to their children, are closest to my heart.

For those parents who read this book, I hope you will have the same trust for the future of your family as my mother does. There are so many other people in your community who are there to support you in your parenting. Not everything is on your shoulders. So many parents have trusted me with their families and for this I will be forever grateful.

As for your own parenting choices, remember you just have to be this side of good enough.

RESOURCE LIST FOR PARENTS

Borba, Michele. *Thrivers: The Surprising Reasons Why Some Kids Struggle and Others Shine*. New York: G.P. Putnam's Sons, 2021.

Brooks, Robert, and Sam Goldstein. *Raising Resilient Children: Fostering Strength, Hope, and Optimism in Your Child*. New York: McGraw Hill, 2002.

Brooks, Robert, and Sam Goldstein. *Tenacity in Children: Nurturing the Seven Instincts for Lifetime Success*. New York: Springer, 2021.

Brown, Brené. *Dare to Lead: Brave Work. Tough Conversations. Whole Hearts*. New York: Random House, 2018.

Fisher, Max. *The Chaos Machine: The Inside Story of How Social Media Rewired Our Minds and Our World*. New York: Little, Brown and Company, 2022.

Knippenberg, Craig. *Legit Parenting* (podcast). https://podcasts.apple.com/us/podcast/legit-parenting/id1557718192.

Knippenberg, Craig. *Wired and Connected: Brain-Based Solutions to Ensure Your Child's Social and Emotional Success*. Littleton, CO: Illumify Media Global, 2019.

Lukianoff, Greg and Jonathan Haidt. *The Coddling of the American Mind: How Good Intentions and Bad Ideas Are Setting Up a Generation for Failure.* New York: Penguin Books, 2018.

Race, Kristen. *Mindful Life* (website). https://mindfullifetoday.com/.

Race, Kristen. *Mindful Parenting: Simple and Powerful Solutions for Raising Creative, Engaged, Happy Kids in Today's Hectic World.* New York: St. Martin's Griffin, 2013.

Setiya, Kieran. *Life Is Hard: How Philosophy Can Help Us Find Our Way.* New York: Riverhead Books, 2022.

Skenazy, Lenore. *Let Grow* (website). https://letgrow.org/.

Spock, Benjamin. *The Common Sense Book of Baby and Child Care.* New York: Duell, Sloan and Pearce, 1946.

Swanson, James M. *School-Based Assessments and Interventions for ADD Students.* Madison, CT: K.C. Publishing, 1992.

Winnicott, Donald W. *Playing and Reality*, 2nd ed. London: Routledge Classics, 2005. First published 1971 by Tavistock Publications Ltd.

NOTES

Introduction

1. Rachel Minkin and Juliana Menasce Horowitz, "Parenting in America Today," Pew Research Center, January 24, 2023, https://www.pewresearch.org/social-trends/2023/01/24/parenting-in-america-today/.

2. D. W. Winnicott, *Playing and Reality*, 2nd edition (London: Routledge Classics, 2005), first published in the UK by Travistock Publications Ltd., 1971.

3. Russell Barkley, "ADHD and the Nature of Self-Control," [presentation], CHADD Annual International Conference on ADHD, 1997, San Antonio, TX.

4. Nataria T. Joseph, Theresa de los Santos, and Lauren Amaro, "Naturalistic Social Cognitive and Emotional Reactions to Technology-mediated Social Exposures and Cortisol in Daily Life," *Biological Psychology* 173 (September 2022), https://doi.org/10.1016/j.biopsycho.2022.108402.

5. Julie Jargon, "The Research Is In: Facebook Mom Groups Really Do Stress Women Out," *The Wall Street Journal*, December 10, 2022,

https://www.wsj.com/articles/the-research-is-in-facebook-mom-groups-really-do-stress-women-out-11670634950.

Chapter 1: It's Okay to Lose It

1. William A. Haseltine, "Depression and Anxiety Double in Youth Compared to Pre-pandemic," *Forbes*, August 24, 2021, https://www.forbes.com/sites/williamhaseltine/2021/08/25/depression-and-anxiety-double-in-youth-compared-to-pre-pandemic/?sh=46b503a0139f.

2. Sam Tabachnik, "Youth Mental Health 'State of Emergency' Is Declared," *The Denver Post*, May 26, 2021.

3. This is also true for your children. A thorough explanation of how to talk to your children when under stress can be found in my first book, *Wired and Connected*.

4. Jessica Grose, "Mother's Little Helper Is Back, and Daddy Is Partaking, Too," *The Denver Post*, October 15, 2020.

5. Brené Brown, *Dare to Lead: Brave Work. Tough Conversations. Whole Hearts* (New York: Random House, 2018), 215.

6. Craig Knippenberg, "An Interview with Whitney Archibald, host of *How She Moms* Podcast," *Legit Parenting* (podcast), December 11, 2021, https://podcasts.apple.com/us/podcast/legit-parenting/id1557718192.

7. Elizabeth A. Stormshak, Karen L. Bierman, Robert J. McMahon, and Liliana J. Lengua, "Parenting Practices and Child Disruptive Behavior Problems in Early Elementary School," *Journal of Clinical Child Psychology* 29, no. 1 (April 2000): 17–29. doi:10.1207/S15374424jccp2901_3.

8. Kristen Race, "The Foundations of Mindful Life Parenting Give YOU the Tools to," accessed June 9, 2023, https://mindfullifetoday.com/foundations-mindful-parenting-course/.

9. Frances E.M. Gardner, "Inconsistent Parenting: Is There Evidence for a Link with Children's Conduct Problems?" *Journal of Abnormal Child Psychology* 17, no. 2 (April 1989): 223–233. doi:10.1007/BF00913796.

Chapter 3: Structure Is Your Friend

1. Jason M. Watson and David L. Strayer, "Supertaskers: Profiles in Extraordinary Multitasking Ability," *Psychonomic Bulletin & Review* 17, no. 4 (August 2010): 479–485. doi:10.3758/PBR.17.4.479. See also Douglas Main, "2 Percent of People Can Multitask Well. Are You a Supertasker?" *Popular Science*, May 9, 2014, https://www.popsci.com/article/science/2-percent-people-can-multitask-well-are-you-supertasker/.

2. Jackie Mader, "Want Resilient and Well-Adjusted Kids? Let Them Play," *The Hechinger Report*, November 14, 2022, https://hechingerreport.org/want-resilient-and-well-adjusted-kids-let-them-play/. See also Jon Hamilton, "Scientists Say Child's Play Helps Build a Better Brain," *NPR Ed, National Public Radio*, August 6, 2014, http://www.npr.org/sections/ed/2014/08/06/336361277/scientists-say-childs-play-helps-build-a-better-brain.

3. Hamilton, "Scientists Say Child's Play Helps Build a Better Brain."

4. Hamilton, "Scientists Say Child's Play Helps Build a Better Brain."

5. Stephanie Granada, "From the Outside In," *Experience Life*, 20, no. 5 (2018): 56.

6. Rob Dunn, "Play Dirty," *Men's Health*, March 2017, 111.

7. Nancy Gibbs, "The Growing Backlash Against Overparenting," *Time*, November 30, 2009, http://content.time.com/time/magazine/article/0,9171,1940697,00.html. See also Hillary L. Burdette and Robert C. Whitaker, "Resurrecting Free Play in Young Children: Looking Beyond Fitness and Fatness to Attention, Affiliation, and Affect," *The Archives of Pediatrics & Adolescent Medicine* 159, no. 1 (2005): 46-50.

8. David Bornstein, "Hard Times for Recess," *The New York Times*, April 4, 2011, https://archive.nytimes.com/opinionator.blogs.nytimes.com/2011/04/04/hard-times-for-recess/.

9. Joe Pinsker, "The Cult of Homework," *The Atlantic*, March 28, 2019, https://www.theatlantic.com/education/archive/2019/03/homework-research-how-much/585889/.

10. Stephen Dubner, "The Economist's Guide to Parenting (Rebroadcast)," *Freakonomics* (podcast), July 5, 2018, http://freakonomics.com/podcast/the-economists-guide-to-parenting-rebroadcast/.

11. See https://letgrow.org/ for more information. The website boldly states, "Treating today's kids as physically and emotionally fragile is bad for their future—and ours. Let Grow counters the culture of overprotection. We aim to future-proof our kids, and our country."

Chapter 4: Structured Gaming

1. Matt Richtel, "Children's Screen Time Has Soared in the Pandemic, Alarming Parents and Researchers," *The New York Times*, January 17, 2021, https://www.nytimes.com/2021/01/16/health/covid-kids-tech-use.html.

2. Richtel, "Children's Screen Time."

3. Veeral Desai, Arnay Gupta, Lucas Andersen, Bailey Ronnestrand, and Michael Wong, "Stress-Reducing Effects of Playing a Casual Video Game among Undergraduate Students," *Trends in Psychology* 29, no. 3 (March 2021): 563–579. doi:10.1007/s43076-021-00062-6.

4. Bingqing Wang, Laramie Taylor, and Qiusi Sun, "Families that Play Together Stay Together: Investigating Family Bonding Through Video Games," *New Media & Society* 20, no. 11 (April 2018): 4074–4094. https://doi.org/10.1177/14614448187676.

5. Michael Rich, interview by Nathan Heffel, "Worried About Your Kid's Smartphone Use? Start Them On A Flip Phone, Plus More Advice," *Colorado Matters*, Colorado Public Radio, August 1, 2018, https://www.cpr.org/news/story/worried-about-your-kids-smartphone-usage-start-them-on-flip-phones-and-more-advice.

6. Kent C. Berridge and Morten L. Kringelbach, "Pleasure Systems in the Brain," *Neuron* 86, no. 3 (May 2015): 646–664. doi:10.1016/j.neuron.2015.02.018.

7. Julie Jargon, "Your Brain's Online Time Warp," *The Wall Street Journal*, January 17, 2023, print edition.

8. Rich, interview by Nathan Heffel, "Worried About Your Kid's Smartphone Use?"
9. Julie Jargon, "Keep Control of Screen Time," *The Wall Street Journal*, September 6, 2022, print edition.

Chapter 5: TikTok Generation

1. U.S. Department of Health and Human Services, *Social Media and Youth Mental Health: The U.S. Surgeon General's Advisory*, 2023, 6, https://www.hhs.gov/surgeongeneral/priorities/youth-mental-health/social-media/index.html.
2. Esteban Ortiz-Ospina, "The Rise of Social Media," Our World in Data (website), September 18, 2019, https://ourworldindata.org/rise-of-social-media.
3. Jenny Brundin, "Colorado Teens Say School Stress, Phones, Social Pressure Are Behind Growing Mental Health Issues," *CPR News*, October 24, 2019. https://www.cpr.org/2019/10/24/colorado-teens-say-school-stress-phones-social-pressure-are-behind-growing-mental-health-issues/.
4. Royal Society for Public Health, "Instagram Ranked Worst for Young People's Mental Health," May 19, 2017, https://www.rsph.org.uk/about-us/news/instagram-ranked-worst-for-young-people-s-mental-health.html.
5. Nirmita Panchal, Heather Saunders, Robin Rudowitz, and Cynthia Cox, "The Implications of COVID-19 for Mental Health and Substance Use," *Kaiser Family Foundation* (KFF), March 20, 2023. https://www.kff.org/coronavirus-covid-19/issue-brief/the-implications-of-covid-19-for-mental-health-and-substance-use/.
6. Carlos Monkus, "CU Boulder Study Shows Screen Time for Children Should Not Worry Parents," *The Denver Post*, December 6, 2020, https://www.denverpost.com/2020/12/06/screen-time-kids-parents-cu-boulder/.
7. Amanda C. Perkovich, *The Impact of Social Media on Teenage Females Self-Esteem* [Master's alternative plan paper], Cornerstone: A Collection of Scholarly and Creative Works for Minnesota State University, Mankato, April 14, 2021. https://cornerstone.lib.mnsu.edu/etds/1104/.

8. Larry Greenemeier, "False News Travels 6 Times Faster on Twitter than Truthful News," *Scientific American*, March 9, 2018, https://www.pbs.org/newshour/science/false-news-travels-6-times-faster-on-twitter-than-truthful-news. See also The Social Institute (website), https://thesocialinstitute.com/understanding-deepfakes-equip-students-to-spot-misinformation-on-social-media-pinterest/.

9. Sara C. Hitchman, Geoffrey T. Fong, Mark P. Zanna, James F. Thrasher, and Fritz L. Laux, "The Relation between Number of Smoking Friends, and Quit Intentions, Attempts, and Success: Findings from the International Tobacco Control (ITC) Four Country Survey," *Psychology of Addictive Behaviors* 28, no. 4 (December 2014): 1144–1152. https://doi.org/10.1037/a0036483.

10. Ira Flatow, "Inside the 'Chaos Machine' of Social Media," *Science Friday* (podcast), March 3, 2023, https://www.sciencefriday.com/segments/the-chaos-machine-social-media/.

11. Flatow, "Inside The 'Chaos Machine.'"

12. Flatow, "Inside The 'Chaos Machine.'"

13. Flatow, "Inside The 'Chaos Machine.'"

14. Stephen M. Kosslyn and G. Wayne Miller, "A New Map of How We Think: Top Brain/Bottom Brain," *The Wall Street Journal*, October 20, 2013, https://www.wsj.com/articles/a-new-map-of-how-we-think-top-brainbottom-brain-1382140494.

15. Dominic Hernandez, "Why Are More Children Going Through Puberty at a Younger Age?" *Texas A&M Today*, January 11, 2018, https://today.tamu.edu/2018/01/11/why-are-more-children-going-through-puberty-at-a-younger-age/.

16. Jo Anne Hubert, "Parents Often Bring Children to Psychiatric ERs to Calm Them, Study Reveals," *Parent Herald*, December 28, 2022, https://www.parentherald.com/articles/109287/20221228/parents-bring-children-psychiatric-ers-calm-study-reveals.htm.

17. Serena Dai, "Looking at Adorable Baby Animals Improves Productivity," *The Atlantic*, October 1, 2012, https://www.theatlantic.com/national/archive/2012/10/looking-adorable-baby-animals-improves-productivity/323047/.

18. See https://trovaofficial.com/ for more information.

19. Craig Knippenberg, "Influencing positive digital habits in a social world. Your game plan to help your kids go pro!" *Legit Parenting* (podcast), April 5, 2022, https://podcasts.apple.com/us/podcast/influencing-positive-digital-habits-in-a-social/id1557718192?i=1000556310725.

20. Craig Knippenberg, "Before the storm...the importance of taking care of your mental health before it becomes a crisis," *Legit Parenting* (podcast), June 21, 2022, https://podcasts.apple.com/us/podcast/before-the-storm-the-importance-of-taking-care/id1557718192?i=1000575533399.

Chapter 6: Validating Emotions

1. John Woodrow Cox, Steven Rich, Linda Chong, John Muyskens, and Monica Ulmanu, "More Than 356,000 Students Have Experienced Gun Violence at School since Columbine," *The Washington Post*, accessed May 30, 2023, https://www.washingtonpost.com/education/interactive/school-shootings-database/.

2. U.S. Congress, Office of Technology Assessment, "Chapter 3: Injury to Students in School," in *Risks to Students in School*, OTA-ENV-633 (Washington, DC: U.S. Government Printing Office, September 1995), 47–114. https://www.princeton.edu/~ota/disk1/1995/9538/953805.PDF.

3. Markian Hawryluk, "As Colorado Reels From another School Shooting, Study Finds 1 in 4 Teens Have Quick Access to Guns," *Colorado Newsline*, March 28, 2023, https://coloradonewsline.com/2023/03/28/colorado-school-shooting-teens-access-guns/.

4. Vivian Yee and Alan Blinder, "National School Walkout: Thousands Protest Against Gun Violence Across the U.S.," *New York Times*, March 14, 2018, https://www.nytimes.com/2018/03/14/us/school-walkout.html.

5. Teresa M. Walker, "League Suspends Ja Morant 25 Games Over Flashing Gun," *The Denver Post*, June 17, 2023, print edition.

6. Max Roser and Hannah Ritchie, "Homicides," *Our World in Data* (December 2019), https://ourworldindata.org/homicides. See also *The*

Roanoke Times, "Prehistoric Violence Worse than Today's," May 31, 1994, https://scholar.lib.vt.edu/VA-news/ROA-Times/issues/1994/rt9405/940531/05310011.htm.

Chapter 7: Validating Emotions: Long-Term Stress

1. Andrea Petersen, "The Pandemic's Terrible Toll on Kids," *Wall Street Journal*, April 9, 2021. https://www.wsj.com/livecoverage/covid-2021-04-09/card/keL7waEBXAb0MfwYxzl2.

2. National Public Radio, "The Kids Aren't Alright: The Post-Pandemic Teen Mental Health Crisis," March 1, 2023, https://www.npr.org/2023/03/01/1160478454/the-kids-arent-alright-the-post-pandemic-teen-mental-health-crisis.

3. Nirmita Panchal, Heather Saunders, Robin Rudowitz, and Cynthia Cox, "The Implications of COVID-19 for Mental Health and Substance Use," *Kaiser Family Foundation* (KFF), March 20, 2023, https://www.kff.org/coronavirus-covid-19/issue-brief/the-implications-of-covid-19-for-mental-health-and-substance-use/. See also Wesley J. Park and Kristen A. Walsh, "COVID-19 and the Unseen Pandemic of Child Abuse," *BMJ Pediatrics Open* (May 2022), https://bmjpaedsopen.bmj.com/content/bmjpo/6/1/e001553.full.pdf.

4. Samantha Laine Perfas, "Young People Are Hurting, and Their Parents Are Feeling It," *The Harvard Gazette*, March 6, 2023, https://news.harvard.edu/gazette/story/2023/03/worried-about-childs-mental-health-youre-not-alone/.

5. Centers for Disease Control and Prevention, "Fast Facts: Preventing Adverse Childhood Experiences," last revised June 29, 2023, https://www.cdc.gov/violenceprevention/aces/fastfact.html.

6. Lauren Camera, "Pandemic Prompts Historic Decline in Student Achievement on Nation's Report Card," *U.S. News & World Report*, October 24, 2022, https://www.usnews.com/news/education-news/articles/2022-10-24/pandemic-prompts-historic-decline-in-student-achievement-on-nations-report-card.

7. Jenny Brundin, "Colorado Teens Say School Stress, Phones, Social Pressure Are Behind Growing Mental Health Issues," *CPR News*, October 24, 2019, https://www.cpr.org/2019/10/24/colorado-teens-say-school-stress-phones-social-pressure-are-behind-growing-mental-health-issues/.

8. Maya L. Rosen, Alexandra M. Rodman, Steven W. Kasparek, Makeda Mayes, Malila M. Freeman, Liliana J. Lengua, Andres N. Meltzoff, Katie A. McLaughlin, "Promoting Youth Mental Health During the COVID-19 Pandemic: A Longitudinal Study," *PLOS ONE* 16, no. 8 (August 11, 2021). https://doi.org/10.1371/journal.pone.0255294.

9. Rachel Feltman, "Worrying You Might Get Hurt Is Worst Than Knowing You Will, Study Finds," *The Washington Post*, March 29, 2016, https://www.washingtonpost.com/news/speaking-of-science/wp/2016/03/29/study-worrying-you-might-get-hurt-is-worse-than-knowing-you-will/.

10. James M. Swanson, *School-Based Assessments and Interventions for ADD Students*, (Madison, CT: K.C. Publishing, 1992), 122.

11. Michael Barbaro, "A Day at the Food Pantry," *The Daily* (podcast), November 11, 2020, https://www.nytimes.com/2020/11/25/podcasts/the-daily/new-york-city-food-pantries.html?showTranscript=1.

Chapter 8: Finding a Purpose

1. Robert Brooks, *The Self-Esteem Teacher* (Loveland, OH: Treehaus Communications, 1991), 31–32.

2. See https://letgrow.org/ for more information.

Chapter 9: Adventures

1. Kyle Benson, "The Magic Relationship Ratio, According to Science," *The Gottman Institute* (website), accessed June 9, 2023, https://www.gottman.com/blog/the-magic-relationship-ratio-according-science/.

Chapter 10: Volunteerism

1. Julie Stevens, "Parent Tips: Integrity," *CSEE Connections* 42, no. 2 (Winter 2022): 28.

Chapter 11: What Do You Want to Keep from Hardship?

1. Lauren Camera, "Pandemic Prompts Historic Decline in Student Achievement on Nation's Report Card," *U.S. News & World Report*, October 24, 2022. https://www.usnews.com/news/education-news/articles/2022-10-24/pandemic-prompts-historic-decline-in-student-achievement-on-nations-report-card.

2. Krista K. Westrick-Payne and Wendy D. Manning, "Marriage, Divorce, and the COVID-19 Pandemic in the U.S.," *Family Profile,* no. 12, 2022. https://www.bgsu.edu/ncfmr/resources/data/family-profiles/westrick-payne-manning-marriage-divorce-covid-pandemic-fp-22-12.html. See also Krista K. Westrick-Payne, Wendy D. Manning, and Lisa Carlson, "Pandemic Shortfall in Marriages and Divorces in the United States," *Socius* 8, November 8, 2022. https://journals.sagepub.com/doi/10.1177/23780231221090192.

3. Brenda K. Wiederhold, "How COVID Has Changed Online Dating—And What Lies Ahead," *Cyberpsychology, Behavior, and Social Networking* 24, no. 7 (July 15, 2021): 435–436. http://doi.org/10.1089/cyber.2021.29219.editorial.

4. Meg Wingerter, "Colorado Teen Drug, Alcohol, and Nicotine Use May Have Fallen During Pandemic, Survey Finds," *The Denver Post*, July 3, 2021, https://www.denverpost.com/2021/07/03/teen-drug-use-colorado-covid-pandemic/.

5. Michele Borba, "Hidden Dangers of Helicopter Parenting," *Michele Borba Ed.D.* (blog), July 16, 2010, https://micheleborba.com/the-big-book-of-parenting-solutions/michele-borba-could-you-be-a-helicopter-parent/.

6. Craig Knippenberg, "Special Guest, Michele Borba Ed D with Craig Knippenberg, LCSW, M.Div. *Thrivers: The Surprising Reasons Why Some Kids Struggle and Others Shine*," *Legit Parenting* (podcast), October 16,

2021, https://podcasts.apple.com/us/podcast/special-guest-michele-borba-ed-d-with-craig/id1557718192?i=1000538780484.

7. Children's Hospital Colorado, "Children's Hospital Colorado Declares a 'State of Emergency' for Youth Mental Health," May 26, 2021, https://www.childrenscolorado.org/about/news/2021/may-2021/youth-mental-health-state-of-emergency/.

8. Jennifer A. Frey, "'Life Is Hard' Review: Suffering Gladly," *The Wall Street Journal*, November 10, 2022, https://www.wsj.com/articles/life-is-hard-review-suffering-gladly-11668122728.

9. Travis Brownley, "The Necessity of Stress," *Heads and Tales at Marin Academy*, December 12, 2013, https://travisma.wordpress.com/2013/12/12/the-necessity-of-stress/.

10. Michael Jordan, "Michael Jordan 'Failure' Commercial HD 1080p," Scott Cole, December 8, 2012, YouTube video, 0:33, https://www.youtube.com/watch?v=JA7G7AV-LT8.

INDEX

Index

ABOUT THE AUTHOR

Craig A. Knippenberg, LCSW, M.Div., founded one of Colorado's largest private mental health practices specializing in child, adolescent, and family development. He also earned notoriety for creating the CONNECT Social Skills Group Program forty years ago. CONNECT has helped thousands of children grow and mature.

Knippengerg is the senior mental health consultant for St. Anne's Episcopal School in Denver. He is the author of *Wired and Connected: Brain-Based Solutions To Ensure Your Child's Social and Emotional Success,* which is based on his social brain curriculum for K-8 students. He is also the host of a popular parenting podcast called *Legit Parenting,* which is available on Apple and Spotify. Find more information about Craig's books, podcast and educational consultation services at Legitparenting.com. He has also authored *I was a Turtle,* which details his emotional experiences from growing up with dyslexia and *Crying for Columbine,* which recounts his experiences as a mental health first responder at the Columbine tragedy.

In 2008, Knippenberg received Denver's Minoru Yasui Volunteer Award for his commitment to mental health consumers. He also was a recipient of the Heroes in the Fight Award from NAMI in 2009. He has served on numerous nonprofit boards that support neurodiverse populations, education, and adoption.

Knippenberg and his son launched AdventureDad.org, a website and blog dedicated to helping dads connect with their kids through adventure.

Printed in the USA
CPSIA information can be obtained
at www.ICGtesting.com
JSHW082202171023
50358JS00010B/37